100 Questions & Answers About Chronic Pain

Vladimir Maletic, MD, MS

Clinical Professor of Neuropsychiatry and Behavioral Science
University of South Carolina School of Medicine
Columbia, South Carolina
Consulting Associate in the Division of Child and Adolescent Psychiatry
Department of Psychiatry
Duke University
Durham, North Carolina

Rakesh Jain, MD, MPH

Director, Adult and Child Psychopharmacology Research
R/D Clinical Research, Inc.
Lake Jackson, Texas
Assistant Clinical Professor
Department of Psychiatry
Texas Tech University Health Science Center
School of Medicine
Lubbock, Texas

Charles L. Raison, MD

Associate Professor, Department of Psychiatry and Behavioral Sciences
Emory University School of Medicine
Atlanta, Georgia

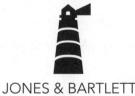

JONES & BARTLETT
LEARNING

World Headquarters

Jones & Bartlett Learning	Jones & Bartlett Learning	Jones & Bartlett Learning
40 Tall Pine Drive	Canada	International
Sudbury, MA 01776	6339 Ormindale Way	Barb House, Barb Mews
978-443-5000	Mississauga, Ontario L5V 1J2	London W6 7PA
info@jblearning.com	Canada	United Kingdom
www.jblearning.com		

Jones & Bartlett Learning books and products are available through most bookstores and online booksellers. To contact Jones & Bartlett Learning directly, call 800-832-0034, fax 978-443-8000, or visit our website, www.jblearning.com.

The authors, editor, and publisher have made every effort to provide accurate information. However, they are not responsible for errors, omissions, or for any outcomes related to the use of the contents of this book and take no responsibility for the use of the products and procedures described. Treatments and side effects described in this book may not be applicable to all people; likewise, some people may require a dose or experience a side effect that is not described herein. Drugs and medical devices are discussed that may have limited availability controlled by the Food and Drug Administration (FDA) for use only in a research study or clinical trial. Research, clinical practice, and government regulations often change the accepted standard in this field. When consideration is being given to use of any drug in the clinical setting, the healthcare provider or reader is responsible for determining FDA status of the drug, reading the package insert, and reviewing prescribing information for the most up-to-date recommendations on dose, precautions, and contraindications, and determining the appropriate usage for the product. This is especially important in the case of drugs that are new or seldom used.

Production Credits
Executive Publisher: Christopher Davis
Editorial Assistant: Sara Cameron
Associate Production Editor: Leah Corrigan
Associate Marketing Manager: Katie Hennessey
Manufacturing and Inventory Control Supervisor: Amy Bacus
Composition: Glyph International
Cover Design: Colleen Lamy
Cover Images: (top) © Photodisc, (bottom left) © Stanislav Fridkin/ShutterStock, Inc.,
  (bottom right) © Minh Tang/Dreamstime.com
Printing and Binding: Malloy, Inc.
Cover Printing: Malloy, Inc.

Library of Congress Cataloging-in-Publication Data
Maletic, Vladimir.
  100 questions & answers about chronic pain/Vladimir Maletic, Rakesh Jain, Charles L. Raison.
    p. cm.
  Includes index.
  ISBN 978-0-7637-8604-5 (alk. paper)
  1. Chronic pain—Popular works. 2. Chronic pain—Miscellanea. I. Jain, Rakesh K. II. Raison, Charles L. III. Title. IV. Title: One hundred questions and answers about chronic pain.
  RB127.M3453 2012
  616'.0472—dc22
                        2010042944

6048

Printed in the United States of America
14 13 12 11 10   10 9 8 7 6 5 4 3 2 1

I wish to dedicate this book to my mother Mara, son Stefan, and wife Marjorie. Without their love, support, and sacrifice, my work on this book would not have been possible.

Vladimir Maletic, MD, MS

I dedicate this book to my parents, Mrs. and Dr. Jain; and to my siblings, Shilpa and Shailesh, whose unwavering support over the years has been the bedrock of my life. I also dedicate this book to my wife, Saundra, for offering me love and encouragement with amazing, unrestrained abundance.

Rakesh Jain, MD, MPH

This book would not have been possible without the constant and ongoing support of my wife, Anne Raison, with more than a little help from my step daughter, Madeleine Stickland.

Charles L. Raison, MD

Contents

Chronic pain is a health problem of awe-inspiring negative power. It causes immeasurable suffering for countless millions of our fellow human beings, and if untreated, it can break the will and spirit of even the strongest man and woman.

In short, chronic pain demands our respect.

We three authors grudgingly respect its terrible power to destroy everything we hold dear. So, although we consider chronic pain a worthy adversary, we believe that it is often a conquerable and controllable problem.

However, a major barrier in chronic pain management is the lack of easily available information to the most important person in the chronic pain equation—the individual with chronic pain. This is the reason we have written this book. Our only intention is to provide you with information and support as you navigate the complexities involved in coming to understand—and access help for—chronic pain. "Chronic pain" is, of course, an umbrella term that covers scores of conditions that cause pain. Each of these is different. They may have different causes, different provocateurs, and different treatments. Those people with chronic pain need to be aware of these issues if they are to become well-informed partners in the treatment process.

This issue of increased knowledge is not optional; it is a must. Study after study reveals the same thing—the informed consumer of medical services gets the best care. This too, is a well-known fact: Chronic pain is not a well-controlled condition in the United States, or for that matter, anywhere in the world. Every journey begins with the first step—we strongly believe that the first step to optimally coping with chronic pain is to become educated about it.

The very fact that this book is in your hands testifies to the interest you have in this issue. This book is intended to offer you a solid knowledge base regarding multiple topics on chronic pain. Several of your questions are answered here: What causes abnormal pain? What goes wrong in the body? What are the chemical and psychological issues at play in chronic pain? Who should I approach in order to get help? What questions should I ask? What are my treatment options? What are the benefits and risks of these treatments? How do I cope with chronic pain?

Are these not the very questions you have? In the decades that the three of us have worked with patients, these and many more are the questions we have heard again and again. You have a right to straightforward, honest, and informative answers. We hope this book answers your questions and that you get maximum relief from your chronic pain. In addition to merely informing you, we wish to offer you our encouragement and support. Progress in chronic pain research and clinical practice is occurring rapidly, and we genuinely and sincerely hope you will get the relief you deserve.

Best of luck, and we hope you benefit from the information in this book.

Vladimir Maletic, MD, MS
Rakesh Jain, MD, MPH
Charles L. Raison, MD

Chronic pain is a very common condition that is often very challenging to manage. Patients suffering from chronic pain could benefit substantially from more education on its mechanisms, daily toll on their lives, and best strategies to manage it. Such pain is also very frequently accompanied by psychiatric conditions, including depression and anxiety disorders, which makes management more difficult and treatment less successful.

This volume, written by Drs. Vladimir Maletic, Rakesh Jain, and Charles L. Raison, provides a very unique resource for patients suffering from chronic pain. Its format is unique and greatly useful as it focuses on the 100 most relevant questions that such patients would ask. It is the result of years of clinical expertise on the topic from the three coauthors, who are greatly experienced psychiatrists with very significant expertise in managing pain conditions. Its down-to-earth, straightforward, patient-oriented approach should be a great strength for patients wanting to learn more about their condition. We are all fortunate to have such a wonderful new resource to recommend to patients suffering from chronic pain, as well as their friends and relatives who could benefit from such information.

Jair C. Soares, MD
Professor and Chairman
Co-Director, University of Texas Center of
Excellence on Mood Disorders
Department of Psychiatry and Behavioral Sciences
University of Texas Medical School at Houston

PART ONE

Introduction to Pain and Pain Disorders

What is pain, and why do we hurt? Can pain sometimes be good?

My spouse has recently been diagnosed with neuropathic pain disorder. Is this a common disease? Can you help me understand it better?

How is fibromyalgia diagnosed?

More . . .

1. What is pain, and why do we hurt? Can pain sometimes be good?

Pain can be defined as an unpleasant sensory, emotional, and cognitive experience generated in response to actual or potential tissue injury. We can immediately appreciate the complex character of pain if we remember our last paper cut or burns in our mouth after drinking a beverage that was too hot. In addition to the unpleasant sensory experience itself, these types of everyday pain are also associated with strong feelings and thoughts (not always voiced aloud). Thus, sensations of pain can be described by their (A) quality, which can be burning, stabbing, stinging, throbbing, dull, or sharp; (B) intensity, which is often measured on a 1 to 10 scale; (C) location, which can be focal or generalized; and (D) duration, which can be acute (brief) or chronic (enduring).

Pain can be good! In fact, the ability to feel pain is absolutely essential for survival. Rarely, humans who are born without pain sensations nearly all die in childhood from an accumulation of unattended injuries because they are not felt as painful. Pain warns us that danger is afoot and that one's current behavior should be adjusted.

Two examples of pain that can be beneficial are nociceptive and inflammatory pain. **Nociceptive pain** is elicited by mechanical, thermal, or chemical injury to our tissues. In this type of pain, diverse painful signals are converted by nociceptors (sensory nerve endings) into an electrochemical signal, which is then propagated to the dorsal horn of the spinal column and eventually to the pain-processing circuitry in the brain, which provides us with a "comprehensive" pain experience. **Inflammatory pain** typically arises in response

---

Pain

An unpleasant sensory, emotional, and cognitive experience generated in response to actual or potential tissue injury.

Pain can be good! In fact, the ability to feel pain is absolutely essential for survival.

Nociceptive pain

Pain caused by tissue injury. Pain is due to mechanical, thermal, or chemical injury to bodily tissue.

Inflammatory pain

Arises in response to infection, tissue damage, or irritation. When our bodies are exposed to injurious stimuli, they commonly generate an "inflammatory soup," which is a mix of chemicals produced by the injured tissue and our immune cells.

to infection. When our bodies become infected by microorganisms, they commonly generate an "inflammatory soup," a mix of chemicals produced by the injured tissue and our immune cells. This mix includes ions, bradykinins, pro-inflammatory cytokines, prostaglandins, and other chemicals. This "inflammatory soup" washes over sensory nerve endings and produces inflammatory pain as a signal warning us that our bodies are under invasion.

It is hard to argue that pain arising from sunburn, after we step on a thumbtack, or when we have an inflamed tooth is not a useful signal. In all these instances pain is likely to generate adaptive behavior (such as getting out of the sun or inspiring a visit to the dentist) that will spare our tissues and organs further injury. Most "good pain" tends to be acute. If this pain persists, its character frequently changes in maladaptive ways, but that is the topic for one of our next headings.

2. Is chronic pain the same as longer-lasting acute pain or are there other differences?

Although it is unpleasant, **acute pain** is really best understood as an adaptive process that is essential for our survival. It is an appropriate, well-modulated, predictable, warning signal aimed at preserving the integrity of our bodies by preventing more extensive injury to our tissues than has already been experienced. Pain often automatically initiates an adaptive response before we even consciously know what we are doing. For example, we touch a hot stove and our hand is off it before our brains have even begun to fully register how much it hurt. Pain lasts longer than the acute danger, and this is often good for our survival, too. Pain tells us to leave the damaged area alone, not to use it, and to be especially careful about keeping it out of harm's way. In some

Acute pain

Pain caused by tissue injury. Typically ceases once the injury has healed.

uncommon circumstances pain and pleasure may result from the same stimuli. Athletes in training and fans of hot curry will fully appreciate this phenomenon as a powerful example of how painful and pleasurable sensations share certain neurobiological connections.

The imaginary boundary separating acute and chronic pain is an arbitrary one. Most often acute pain does not last longer than a month or two (e.g., pain associated with the healing of a broken bone). Once the healing process is complete, acute pain spontaneously decreases. On the other hand, chronic pain typically lasts long after healing has occurred. This, in itself, highlights the fact that chronic pain is not just acute pain that lasts longer. While acute pain represents a normal physiologic phenomenon, chronic pain is a manifestation of a deep-rooted disease state. Most often **chronic pain** will persist in the absence of an ongoing stimulus, long after the underlying disease has been treated or cured, sometimes lasting months or even years. Unlike acute pain, which tends to be focused on the site of injury, chronic pain is often diffuse and may have no observable anatomical underpinning. Although there is no agreement about a separation point between acute and chronic pain, pain lasting longer than 3 months is typically considered to be chronic.

Chronic pain is classified as *neuropathic* or *pain of mixed origin* (including some inflammatory and neuropathic components). Unlike acute pain, which originates in damaged tissue, chronic pain is believed to arise from alterations in the function and structure of the central nervous system (i.e., the brain and spinal cord). Chronic pain is a result of the brain misinterpreting, and further amplifying peripheral pain signals. Peripheral and spinal column pain pathways are sensitized

Chronic pain

Persists in the absence of an ongoing stimulus, well beyond the resolution of the underlying disease, sometimes lasting for months or even years.

and magnify incoming pain signals, which the brain processes incorrectly, leading to inappropriate descending pain modulation, thus perpetuating this vicious cycle.

3. When I last visited my doctor, she mentioned peripheral sensitization as one of the causes of my pain. What is that?

Specialized pain-sensing nerve endings, called **nociceptors**, detect chemical, mechanical, or thermal injury to our tissues. After nociceptors convert painful signals into an electrochemical impulse, it is passed on to a nerve cell body situated in the dorsal root ganglia (DRG) of the spinal cord (see **Figure 1**). Departing from the DRG, the pain signal is carried out by lightly myelinated alpha-delta and unmyelinated slow C-fibers to secondary sensory neurons located in the dorsal column. Under usual circumstances, once the harmful stimulus

Nociceptors

Specialized pain-sensing nerve endings that detect chemical, mechanical, or thermal injury to our tissues.

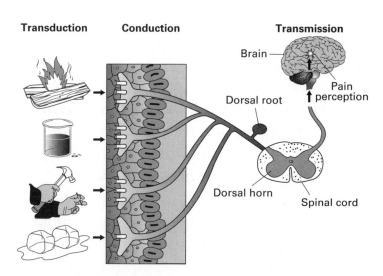

Figure 1   After nociceptors convert painful signals into a neurochemical impulse (transduction), it is passed on to a nerve cell body situated in the dorsal root ganglia (DRG) of the spinal cord (conduction), and then on to the dorsal horn of the spinal cord and the brain (transmission).

Introduction to Pain and Pain Disorders

subsides, the pain transmission stops. Unfortunately, sometimes a different scenario occurs. Painful signals continue to flow from the peripheral nerves to the dorsal column long after the harmful stimulus has stopped or to a degree that is out of proportion to the magnitude of the original source of pain. This magnification process is called **peripheral sensitization**. Here is how it happens.

Peripheral sensitization

Painful signals continue to flow from the periphery to dorsal column, long after the harmful stimulus has stopped or to a degree that is excessively out of proportion to the magnitude of the original source of pain.

Tissue damage may produce an extended inflammatory state. This state can be thought of as an "inflammatory soup" composed of diverse molecules, such as hydrogen ions, adenosine tri-phosphate (ATP), prostaglandins, bradykinins, and pro-inflammatory cytokines. This "soup" washes over nociceptive nerve endings. These signaling molecules bind to receptors on the surface of the nerve cells and activate enzymes within neurons called protein kinases. Activated enzymes interact with ion channels and receptors, changing their signaling properties. The end result of this process is that the threshold for pain neurons to fire goes down so that they fire more easily. Heightened sensitivity of the pain-sensing nerve endings is the hallmark of peripheral sensitization.

4. I am a long time sufferer from neuropathic pain. During my last visit the doctor said that my pain is caused by central sensitization. What is that and how does it happen?

Central sensitization

Magnified pain experience resulting from disrupted pain modulation at several levels of the central nervous system. This type of pain tends to be diffuse and generalized.

Central sensitization is a key feature of chronic pain disorders. Central sensitization results from disrupted pain modulation at several levels of the central nervous system. A number of central nervous system (CNS) areas including dorsal horn neurons, pain-processing areas in the brain (also known as the "pain matrix") and descending pain-modulatory pathways (see **Figure 2**) have all been implicated as the neural foundation of

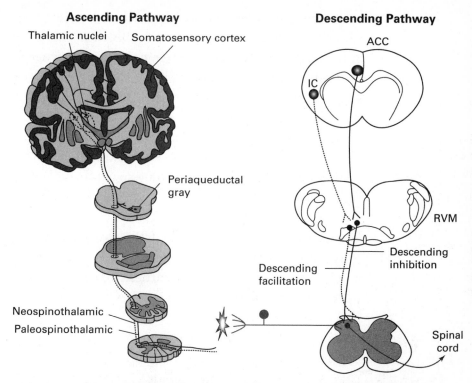

Figure 2   A number of CNS areas including dorsal horn neurons, pain-processing areas in the brain (also known as the "pain matrix"), and descending pain-modulatory pathways have all been implicated as neural underpinning of the aberrant neurotransmission that leads to the development of central sensitization.

ACC = Anterior cingulate cortex, a point of origin for descending pain-enhancing fibers; IC = Insular cortex, origination point for pain-inhibiting fibers; RVM = Rostral ventral medulla, a "hub" for descending pain-modulating fibers.

the aberrant neurotransmission that leads to the development of central sensitization. Unlike peripheral sensitization, where excessive pain remains localized in the injured area, pain tends to be diffuse and generalized in central sensitization.

Heightened dorsal horn excitability can sometimes be caused by increased peripheral nociceptor activity. In this way, peripheral sensitization can contribute to central sensitization. When this happens, overly active pain-receptive nerves release large amounts of pain-signaling molecules, such as glutamate, substance-P (SP), and neurotrophic factors (chemicals that influence nerve-cell branching and resilience). After crossing the synaptic cleft, these neuromodulators bind to their respective receptors, initiating chemical signaling cascades within the cell, eventually activating enzymes called phosphokinases. These enzymes mediate changes in characteristics of receptors and ion channels, making dorsal horn neurons overly sensitive to incoming signals in an enduring manner (see **Figure 3**).

Central sensitization can also be triggered and sustained by stimulation of certain genes, such as the one regulating an enzyme in charge of the synthesis of prostaglandin PGE_2 (one of the chemical mediators of inflammation).

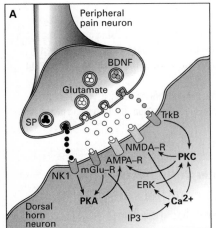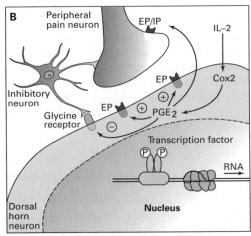

Figure 3   These pain-altered enzymes change characteristics of receptors and ion channels, making dorsal horn neurons overly sensitive to incoming signals in an enduring manner.
Panel A: SP = Substance P, a pain modulator; NK-1 = neurokinin type 1 receptor to which SP attaches; BDNF = Brain-derived neurotrophic factor; TrkB = a type of BDNF receptor; AMPA-R, NMDA-R, and mGlu-R = types of glutamate receptors; PKA and PKC = phosphokinase A and C, enzymes involved in regulation of receptor activity; ERK and IP3 = types of intracellular signaling molecules; Panel B: IL-2 = interleukin-2, an inflammatory molecule; Cox-2 = cyclooxygenase-2, an enzyme involved in synthesis of inflammatory prostaglandins; PGE_2 = prostaglandin E_2, an inflammatory molecule; EP and IP = prostaglandin receptors.

Prostaglandins, in turn, make neurons more excitable. Additionally, central sensitization in neuropathic pain (NeP) may be a consequence of a "short circuit" due to irregular growth of pressure-sensing nerve fibers that form new connections with pain neurons in the dorsal horn. Signals may thus get "mixed up" so that touch and pressure are experienced as pain.

Slow pain-conducting nerve fibers (C-fibers) are also capable of "backward" release of pain transmitters into the injured tissue, which then causes "neurogenic inflammation" (inflammation caused by nerves). This vicious cycle may further enhance chronic pain. Clinical manifestations of central sensitization will be discussed shortly.

5. I read that people suffering from neuropathic pain often have allodynia and hyperalgesia. Could you explain what these are?

People afflicted by neuropathic pain often experience non-painful stimuli such as touch and pressure as pain. This is a phenomenon referred to as **allodynia**. Some chronic painful conditions are associated with **hyperalgesia**, which is a tendency to experience painful stimuli as much more intense than they really are. Very often, individuals suffering from neuropathic pain experience burning and tingling in various parts of their body, also known as **paresthesia**. These clinical features are dramatically disproportionate to the typically very modest physical findings in the areas of pain.

Significant problems in professional, social, and intimate relationships may occur as a result of allodynia and hyperalgesia. The challenge of living with neuropathic pain is often increased by a lack of understanding: how can one experience so much suffering in the

Allodynia

Propensity to experience non-painful stimuli, such as touch and pressure, as pain. Allodynia is a common feature of many chronic pain disorders.

Hyperalgesia

A tendency to experience painful stimuli as much more intense than they really are.

Paresthesia

Altered feeling of pain that can affect any nerve(s) in the body. Patients typically report burning and/or tingling pain.

absence of a visible cause? The answer, of course, is that the pain is real, but it is being produced by pain circuits in the brain rather than at the site where the pain is felt to exist. It is important that health professionals spend some time educating patients and their family members about the impact of these central sensitization-related phenomena.

6. My spouse has recently been diagnosed with neuropathic pain disorder. Is this a common disease? Can you help me understand it better?

Neuropathic pain (NeP)

Typically caused by direct nerve injury or damage to neural tissue, resulting in abnormal sensory processing.

Neuropathic pain (NeP) is typically caused by direct nerve injury or damage to neural tissue, resulting in abnormal sensory processing. NeP is commonly associated with hyperalgesia (increased sensitivity to painful stimuli), allodynia (abnormal pain response to non-noxious stimuli), and paresthesia (spontaneous tingling and burning sensations). NeP is a fairly common condition. Estimates suggest that forms of NeP (diabetic neuropathy, postherpetic neuralgia, trigeminal neuralgia, spinal cord injury, radiculopathy, etc.) affect 26 million people worldwide and approximately 1.5% of the U.S. population. One in four patients in pain clinics suffers from this debilitating and largely treatment-resistant condition. The frequency of NeP varies from country to country for reasons not fully understood. For example, a large United Kingdom survey reported 8% prevalence of pain of predominantly neuropathic origin. On the other hand, an Austrian epidemiologic study found a significantly lower prevalence of NeP (3.3%). Two-thirds of the study sample suffered from pain for longer than a year. Pain tended to be severe, enduring, and associated with significant functional impairment. Like in fibromyalgia, women were more likely to suffer from NeP than men.

7. I recently read about temporal summation of second pain and "windup" in fibromyalgia. Can you explain these events?

Temporal summation of "second pain" (TSSP) is one of the hallmark clinical features of fibromyalgia (FM). TSSP results from constant stimulation of "slow-conducting" C-fibers, which then produces progressive electrical discharges from dorsal horn neurons ("windup"), causing pain. **"First pain,"** which is conducted by "faster" myelinated A-delta fibers, is commonly described as sharp, stabbing, and well-defined. By contrast, "second pain," conveyed by unmyelinated, slow C-fibers, tends to be characterized as dull, aching, burning, and less well-defined. In experimental conditions, second pain rapidly intensifies when painful stimuli are applied with frequency greater than once every 3 seconds. "Temporal summation" refers to a neural tendency to add up rapid, mildly painful impulses and translate them into a more intense painful experience. This phenomenon is considered a basis for widespread central sensitization in FM. Researchers have found that TSSP is associated with increased brain activity in several pain-processing areas in FM patients, compared to healthy individuals. It appears that enhanced pain sensitivity in the context of FM may arise more from altered activity of the entire "pain matrix," rather than from its individual components. These findings have interesting implications, as they suggest that peripheral and central factors "collaborate" in creating the fibromyalgia pain.

8. What is fibromyalgia? Is it just a "fad" or a real disorder?

Fibromyalgia (FM) is, unfortunately, all too real. Although 10% to 12% of the population worldwide and in the United States endure chronic widespread

Temporal summation of "second pain" (TSSP)

This is a complex response whereby pain fibers, when continuously stimulated by pain or inflammation, "learn to over-feel" pain. Intensity of pain is out of proportion with the actual injury, and patients often report dull, aching, burning, and diffuse, spread-out pain. TSSP is associated with elevated activity in several brain pain-processing areas.

"First pain"

Initial pain experience produced by activation of myelinated A-delta type pain fibers. Commonly described as sharp, stabbing, and well-defined.

Fibromyalgia (FM)

Characterized by chronic widespread pain (tenderness in at least 11 of 18 predefined points on the surface of the body), lasting at least 3 months, typically accompanied by fatigue and sleep disturbance.

pain, only about 2% of individuals (3.4% of women and 0.5% of men) meet the American College of Rheumatology (ACR) criteria for FM. The majority of patients with FM are between the ages of 35 to 60 years. Fibromyalgia is characterized by chronic widespread pain (tenderness in at least 11 of 18 predefined points on the surface of the body) lasting at least 3 months, typically accompanied by fatigue and sleep disturbance. Secondary symptoms include morning stiffness and cognitive impairment, often referred to as "fibro-fog." While no single origin has been identified, a unifying theory suggests that FM is a consequence of sensitization of the central nervous system. The onset of fibromyalgia is frequently preceded by a major stressful event, physical trauma, viral illness, catastrophic event (such as war, but not natural disasters), and/or other chronic pain disorders (i.e., osteo- or rheumatoid arthritis). Patients suffering from FM are often afflicted by other medical and psychiatric conditions, such as mood or anxiety disorders, interstitial cystitis, irritable bowel syndrome (IBS), tension headaches, and vulvodynia. Some researchers believe that all these disorders may share pathophysiological mechanisms.

9. How is fibromyalgia diagnosed?

Fibromyalgia is not a fancy name used to describe pain of unknown origin. Contrary to common belief, FM is a well-defined condition, characterized by widespread pain and tenderness impacting all four quadrants of the body, fatigue, and sleep disturbance. Associated symptoms often include depression, anxiety, and problems with thinking. In order to be diagnosed with FM, widespread pain needs to be accompanied by significant functional limitations and last at least 3 months or more. Since various experts in the field held differing opinions, the American College of Rheumatology has put forth its own criteria in order to create a common understanding and facilitate fibromyalgia research. Although ACR criteria were originally designed for research purposes, over time they have become widely used in clinical practice as well. An examination informed by ACR criteria assesses the presence of pain at 18 predefined spots, called "tender points." In addition to the previously outlined criteria, the presence of pressure-provoked pain in 11 out of 18 tender points is diagnostic of FM. A family history of chronic pain disorders, a past medical history of regional pain, psychiatric disorders, or recent stressors should all add to the doctor's suspicion that a patient has FM. If pain symptoms have recent onset, a more intensive testing process may be in order. If the previously mentioned complaints are long-standing, virtually no additional workup is necessary. Nonetheless, at some point most doctors will consider the following labs to assure that other underlying medical conditions are not contributing to symptoms: complete blood count (to rule out anemia); chemistry panel (to evaluate for metabolic disease); thyroid and parathyroid function tests; vitamin D, vitamin B12, and folate levels (to rule out symptoms caused by the lack of vitamins); sedimentation rate; and C-reactive protein. Other tests may be considered if clinically indicated.

10. Why do so many fibromyalgia and neuropathic pain patients also suffer from depression and anxiety?

Many patients suffering from either FM or NeP (or both) will also meet criteria for a major depressive disorder and anxiety disorders. Moreover, patients with FM are at significantly increased risk of developing a depressive disorder and other related psychiatric conditions. For example, an influential study reported that patients with FM were 4.3 times more likely to develop a major depressive disorder at some point in their lives and 4.7 times more likely to develop an anxiety disorder. Overall depression and anxiety are among the most common comorbidities of FM, with frequency ranging from 20% to 80% and 13% to 63.8%. A high comorbidity between depression and pain is not restricted to subjects with FM; it has also been noted in NeP patients. For example, an Austrian epidemiologic study reported depression in 34%, and anxiety in 25%, of NeP patients.

Relationships between major depressive disorders, anxiety disorders, FM, and NeP are complex. It is increasingly apparent that, like major depressive and anxiety disorders, conditions characterized by chronic pain share a progressive course, characterized by altered thought process, as well as structural changes within the brain.

Conditions characterized by chronic pain share a progressive course, characterized by altered thought process, as well as structural changes within the brain.

As noted previously, recent scientific evidence suggests that NeP and FM are characterized by central sensitization. Major depressive disorder is widely considered to be associated with a very similar type of progressive phenomenon known as "kindling." In the context of depression, kindling implies that each episode of depression makes future depressive episodes more likely and less dependent upon external factors such as stress or sickness. Some authors have recently suggested that kindling and sensitization may have similar neurobiological bases, such as lasting changes in the synapse and gene function. Some have even proposed "neurosensitization" as a common origin for chronic pain, depression, and certain anxiety disorders, such as posttraumatic stress disorder (PTSD).

11. Can stress make pain disorders worse?

Fibromyalgia, neuropathic pain, anxiety disorders, and major depression are all either increased or aggravated by stress. In addition to peripheral and central sensitization, FM and NeP are characterized by changes in limbic and cortical functions and the structure in the brain (see **Figure 4**). In addition to managing pain, these limbic and cortical brain areas share many elements with the circuitry involved in stress response and mood regulation. Remarkably, functional imaging studies show that brain areas associated with negative emotional experience in response to physical pain also mediate distress in response to the "pain" of social exclusion. This strongly suggests that emotional and physical pain so often co-occur because they share the same central nervous system networks. Consistent with this, similar functional and structural changes in the brain areas involved with emotional regulation (the amygdala and hippocampus; see **Figure 5**) have been

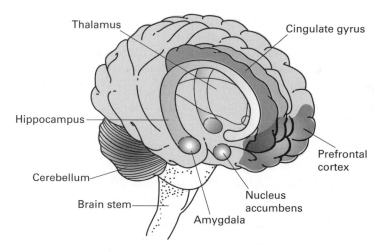

Figure 4   Fibromyalgia (FM) and neuropathic pain (NeP) are characterized by changes in the limbic (amygdala, nucleus accumbens, and hippocampus) and cortical (prefrontal and anterior cingulate cortex) function and structure in the brain.

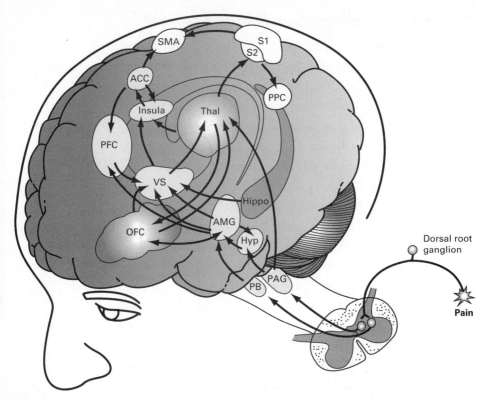

Figure 5   Functional and structural changes in brain areas involved with emotional regulation (amygdala and hippocampus) have been described in chronic stress, major depressive disorders, anxiety disorders, FM, and NeP. The "Pain Matrix," brain areas involved in processing sensory, emotional, and cognitive (thoughts) information related to pain.
ACC = Anterior cingulate cortex; AMG = Amygdala; Hippo = Hippocampus; Hyp = Hypothalamus; Insula = Insular cortex; OFC = Orbitofrontal cortex; PAG = Periaqueductal gray; PB = Parabrachial nucleus; PFC = Prefrontal cortex; SMA = Supplementary motor area; S1, S2 = Somatosensory cortex; Thal = Thalamus; VS = Ventral striatum.

described in chronic stress, major depressive disorders, anxiety disorders, FM, and NeP. Dysfunction of these limbic formations is believed to lead to further disturbances in hormonal, autonomic, and immune functioning, which may further contribute to the worsening of mood and pain symptoms. Additionally, several studies have suggested that the core symptoms of pain disorders (i.e., pain, chronic fatigue, sleep disturbance, and cognitive complaints) significantly complicate the treatment of major depression because these symptoms tend to be especially nonresponsive to conventional treatments. In summary, available evidence suggests that chronic stress, major depression, anxiety disorders, and FM/NeP mutually amplify each other, thus contributing greatly to the treatment burden in depressive, anxiety, and pain disorders.

Sue said:

When I'm stressed or worried, the tension settles in my neck and shoulders. I try to keep my stress in check but that isn't always as easy as it sounds, so I also routinely check how tight my muscles are in my neck and shoulders and then use relaxation exercises to relieve the tension.

Katie said:

During times of intense stress—after my mother's death, when my work schedule gets hectic, or when I have experienced conflicts with my husband, friends, or coworkers, I find myself experiencing more frequent flare-ups of my chronic pain. My entire body hurts. I become exhausted, but I can't sleep. The lack of sleep gives me headaches, stomachaches, and back pain, which, in turn, make it even more difficult for me to sleep. I find myself letting important things slide: I do less at work, I forget appointments and other important events; I don't have the energy to clean the house. I have less patience with my son and become aggravated by little, unimportant things. My husband also has noticed that when I'm stressed I have a tendency to lose things. It has become a signal in my family. When he sees me searching the house for my car keys he tells me to go take a bath or offers to massage my back— anything to help me relax so that I can break the cycle of pain, sleeplessness, and irritation.

12. As a chronic pain sufferer, I often find myself having these three problems: fatigue, trouble sleeping, and memory difficulties. How are they related to my pain?

Bidirectional relationship

Reciprocal relationship. In the context of chronic pain there is an increased risk of sleep, mood, and anxiety disorders in pain sufferers, and vice versa: depression, anxiety, and sleep disturbance predict the development of widespread pain.

Your experience is all too common in individuals suffering from pain. There is a known **bidirectional relationship** between pain and sleep. Individuals with chronic pain conditions tend not to sleep very well. Sleep disruption, in turn, intensifies pain. A recent study of fibromyalgia (FM) patients found a strong relationship between the number of tender points and quality of sleep during the previous night. Patients who slept poorly had a significantly greater number of tender points. Both sleep disorders and chronic pain have also been associated with a decrease in hippocampus gray matter volume. The hippocampus (see Figures 4 and 5) is a brain structure that plays a key role in emotional regulation and stress responses, but also in spatial and declarative memory (i.e., being able to find the right word and remember names). How often has it happened to us that when we are sleep deprived or distressed, we forget where we put things? In similar circumstances one can also have problems articulating thoughts or remembering names. A recent neuroimaging study has found an association between chronic pain and diminished gray matter volume of the dorsolateral prefrontal cortex (DLPFC). Chronic insomnia has also been linked with reduced DLPFC metabolic activity. This is of particular interest since DLPFC has a major role in working memory and effortful sustained attention (see **Figure 6**). Hypothetically, the union of chronic pain and insomnia might have an additional negative impact on memory and thinking. Empirical studies have also highlighted the important role of sleep in memory processes.

Introduction to Pain and Pain Disorders

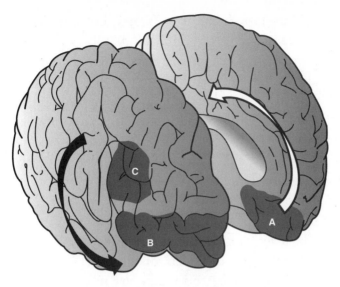

Figure 6 DLPFC has a major role in working memory and effortful sustained attention. A. Ventromedial prefrontal cortex (VMPFC); B. Lateral orbital prefrontal cortex (LOPFC); C. Dorsolateral prefrontal cortex (DLPFC).

Sleep also has an important role in immune regulation. Evidence suggests that sleep deprivation, much like chronic pain, may increase inflammation. We can all recall times when we had a headache and our body felt sore after a sleepless night. Inflammatory cytokines tend to be elevated in patients with sleep disturbance or with chronic pain. Remarkably, they are also elevated in individuals suffering from chronic fatigue. It is plausible to assume that the relationship between sleep disturbance, chronic pain, and memory problems may be controlled at least in part by elevated inflammatory responses and common functional and structural changes in the brain.

Evidence suggests that sleep deprivation, much like chronic pain, may increase inflammation.

Chronic Fatigue Syndrome (CFS)

A prolonged medical condition of unknown cause, characterized by a sensation of exhaustion, inability to carry out physical and intellectual tasks, fever, aches, and depression.

13. Why do chronic fatigue patients so often have pain complaints?

Chronic Fatigue Syndrome (CFS) is a frequently devastating condition characterized by a sensation of exhaustion and inability to carry out physical and intellectual tasks. Once CFS has developed, it tends to be permanent. Despite sustained research efforts, we still do not have laboratory tests capable of confirming CFS nor a clear understanding of its origin and disease process. Viral infections, trauma, and neuroimmune and neuroendocrine factors are all being considered as potential causes of CFS. Autonomic deregulation is a common feature. Frequency estimates range from 0.5% to 2.5% in the general population. It is twice as likely to occur in women as in men. Early manifestations often include fever, upper respiratory and digestive symptoms, muscle aches, sleep disturbance, and fatigue. Rest provides partial and temporary relief, and stress is likely to escalate the symptoms. A seasonal pattern of symptom expression is not uncommon.

Over time, many CFS patients will suffer from headaches, migratory joint pain, generalized muscle aches, sore throat, and chest pain. Patients with CFS typically suffer from a number of other related conditions, including fibromyalgia and mood and anxiety disorders. As in other pain conditions, some studies have found proof that hormonal deregulation and elevated inflammatory and sympathetic responses may contribute to increased pain sensitivity.

14. I heard that childhood trauma is sometimes associated with fibromyalgia and chronic fatigue. Is this true?

Yes, research has found that childhood trauma can be a risk factor for both fibromyalgia and chronic fatigue. To better understand the connection between trauma, CFS, and FM, it may be helpful to go beyond the descriptive classifications of neuropsychiatric disorders and learn about the common underlying disease mechanisms.

Trauma, mood and anxiety disorders, and FM are all associated with brain function disturbance in areas involved in the regulation of emotions, pain, and the stress response. Continuous altered activity in these brain regions will often cause "brain remodeling," or change in the brain structure. More active brain pathways release chemicals called neurotrophic factors, which cause nerve cells to branch out and establish rich connections, while pathways with diminished activity tend to wither away (see **Figure 7**). With time, these changes may become "hardwired," resulting in a loss of adaptive function. Regulation of pituitary and adrenal hormones, sympathetic response, and inflammation are all interrelated and compromised in individuals suffering from post-traumatic stress disorder, depression, FM, and CFS.

As discussed in several other sections of this book, central sensitization—a tendency to respond to painful stimuli with an exaggerated intensity—may be a core

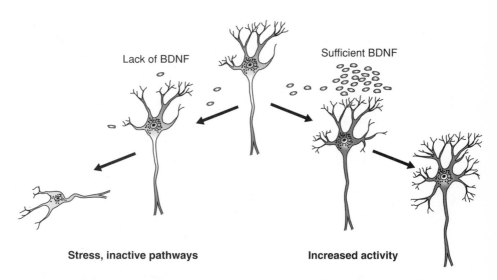

Lack of BDNF

Sufficient BDNF

Stress, inactive pathways

Increased activity

Figure 7 **More active brain pathways release chemicals called neurotrophic factors, which cause nerve cells to branch out and establish rich connections, while pathways with diminished activity tend to wither away.**
BDNF = Brain-derived neurotrophic factor.

manifestation of the shared pathophysiological features of these conditions.

15. I have had painful nodules and spasms in the muscles of my face for several months. My doctor told me that it may be myofascial pain. What is that?

Myofascial pain

A chronic condition associated with localized muscle stiffness and pain (often severe); palpable hypersensitive nodules in muscle tissue, often referred to as "trigger points"; referred tenderness and pain; and motor and autonomic dysfunction. It is believed to be based on central sensitization.

The diagnosis of **myofascial pain** has been a point of heated debate and controversy for several decades. Some researchers consider it to be only a specific manifestation of a greater category of musculoskeletal pain disorders, while others believe that it should be a condition in its own right. It is associated with localized muscle stiffness and pain; palpable hypersensitive nodules in muscle tissue, often referred to as "trigger points"; referred tenderness and pain; motor and autonomic dysfunction; and a phenomenon akin to central sensitization.

Myofascial pain is not an infrequent occurrence. It has been reported in more than 50% of women and more than 40% of men, mostly between the ages of 25 to 50 years. In its active form, pain is continuous, accompanied by stiffness, cramps, muscle weakness, and referred pain in response to direct pressure. In its latent form, there may be occasional cramps, and sharp pain is elicited when pressure is applied. Tension headaches, tearfulness, balance problems, and humming or buzzing in the ears (tinnitus) often accompany myofascial pain. Anxiety, depression, and other chronic pain disorders tend to be associated with myofascial pain syndrome.

The theoretical explanation for the causes of myofascial pain states that nerve fibers in the facial muscles release excessive neurotransmitter acetylcholine initiating the development of myofascial pain. Excessive acetylcholine makes the facial muscles contract, which in turn leads to the release of inflammatory activators that further sensitize the nerve endings. Overly sensitized nerves feed into pain-related brain areas, overwhelming their capacity to process pain signals thus producing a generalized and intensified sensation of myofascial pain .

16. Are myofascial pain and "TMJ" one and the same, or are these two separate conditions?

Although both of these conditions may result in facial pain, **temporomandibular joint (TMJ) pain disorders** and myofascial pain are two different entities. Patients with TMJ usually present with facial pain, limited motion or stiffness in the muscles of the lower jaw, and crackling sounds when making chewing motions. Additionally, patients will often complain of headaches, pain and buzzing in their ears, dizziness, and neck pain. TMJ most often occurs in individuals between the ages of 20 to 50 years. Females are far more likely than males to suffer with TMJ. Indeed, studies report a female to male ratio of from 3:1 to as high as 9:1. In approximately 40% of cases symptoms occur spontaneously, and fortunately, less than 10% of patients require treatment.

TMJ is believed to have complex origins: genetic, environmental, behavioral, and psychosocial factors interact to produce this disorder. Genes that influence the function of brain circuits involved in pain processing have been implicated in conferring vulnerability toward TMJ. Trauma to ligaments, cartilage, and the jaw bone may cause an accumulation of toxic and inflammatory chemicals in the joint tissue. This may lead to functional deterioration and degeneration of the joint and muscle tissue, causing pain. If the pain persists, it may cause changes in pain-controlling circuitry in the brain, leading to central sensitization.

Temporomandibular joint (TMJ) pain disorders

The jaw bone is connected to the skull with a hinge joint. When this joint degenerates or becomes inflamed, a person can experience facial pain, limited motion, or stiffness in the muscles of the lower jaw, and crackling sounds while making chewing motions. Additionally, patients will often complain of headaches, pain and buzzing in their ears, dizziness, and neck pain.

Introduction to Pain and Pain Disorders

23

17. I know that adults can suffer from chronic pain. Can this condition develop in children also?

Yes, unfortunately, children also can develop chronic pain disorders. Several components of the nervous system involved in pain processing, as well as in hormonal and immune response to pain, are still in development in infancy, which makes this age particularly vulnerable to the development of chronic pain conditions. Exposure to repeated or ongoing pain or trauma in this phase of life can have enduring and dramatic effects on the structure and function of developing pain pathways. Hospital procedures, blood sampling, immunizations, prematurity, stress, maternal separation (e.g., a stay in an intensive care unit) all can have a cumulative impact on the brain in this critical period of development and can lead to more than pain sensitization. Indeed, in addition to chronic pain, evidence suggests that childhood pain increases the risk for lasting dysregulation of the immune and endocrine systems. Normal brain development can be disrupted. Pain in childhood has also been linked to impaired wound healing, poor emotional bonding, metabolic disorders, and obesity.

While most children can communicate the presence of pain and even provide simple descriptions of its location, quality, and intensity; infants and toddlers may not be able to do so. In these very young children, pain can be inferred by changes in facial expression, lip pursing, chin quiver, withdrawal of painful part of the body from touch, loud and distressed crying, and changes in sleep and feeding routines. Monitoring observable changes that occur in response to pain, such as pupil dilatation, increased heart rate and blood pressure, palm sweating, flushing, and pallor, can greatly assist with establishing a pain diagnosis. Finally, it is important to recognize that children can develop the same types of pain disorders as adults, including acute and chronic pain.

18. My friend was hit in the head with a bat during a baseball practice. Ten hours later he developed a strong headache and started vomiting. In the ER they told him that he could have died had he not come in. What are these "deadly headaches" all about?

Head trauma can be associated with four types of bleeding or hemorrhage, all accompanied by headache:

1. Intraparenchymal hematoma (a blood clot within the brain) results from bleeding inside the brain tissue itself. The extent of injury depends on the type and caliber of the blood vessel injured, its location, and the composition of the surrounding brain tissue.

2. Epidural (outside the dura) hematoma is often caused by the tear of one of the meningeal arteries, often following a skull fracture. Meninges are membranes surrounding the brain. Dura is a hard membrane next to the skull, and the pia and arachnoid are soft (spiderweb-like) membranes enwrapping the brain and spinal column (see **Figure 8**). Accumulation of blood creates a "pocket" by detaching the dura from the skull. Individuals can be fully conscious for several hours, often complaining of headaches. However, within 6 to 8 hours, dramatic neurological signs usually develop, including abnormal body posture and pupils that are unresponsive to light. Shortly after the development of these signs, the individual typically becomes unconscious and sinks into a coma followed by death.

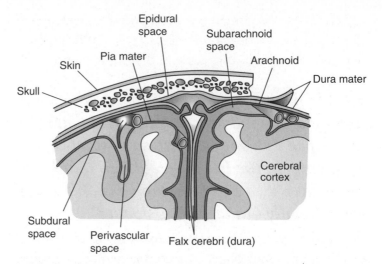

Figure 8 Meninges are membranes surrounding the brain. Dura is a hard membrane next to the skull; the pia and arachnoid are soft (spiderweb-like) membranes enwrapping the brain and spinal column.

3. Subdural (underneath the dura) hematoma is most often caused by a head injury that results in tearing of smaller veins draining the brain. Blood slowly collects in the space between the dura and the brain tissue. Signs and symptoms of subdural hemorrhage include: headache (often fluctuating in intensity), dizziness, blurry vision, loss of appetite, nausea and vomiting, irritability, confusion and disorientation, weakness, numbness, and occasionally seizures. Symptoms usually develop more slowly, usually within 24 hours, although they can sometimes take as long as 2 weeks. Although we cannot be certain based on the brief description, this is the most likely cause of your friend's "deadly headache."

4. Subarachnoid hemorrhage will be discussed in more detail in Question 19. Radiological studies can be used to diagnose and differentiate these intracranial (inside the skull) hemorrhages.

19. My grandfather went to the emergency room because of a severe headache. They told him that he had suffered from a subarachnoid hemorrhage. What is that?

A recent study found that 12% of patients presenting to the emergency room with "the worst headache" they had ever experienced were suffering from a subarachnoid hemorrhage. This highlights how common this condition is and how heightened suspicion and timely diagnosis can be lifesaving.

Subarachnoid hemorrhage is caused by bleeding into the space between the arachnoid membrane and pia mater, which are soft membranes enveloping the brain ("subarachnoid space"). (See the description of meninges in Question 18 and Figure 8.) The hemorrhage is usually caused by spontaneous rupture of a cerebral aneurysm, although occasionally it will follow trauma to the head. Between 20% to 50% of the time, patients report distinct, severe, rapidly developing "thunderclap" headaches. These warning headaches may last from hours to weeks. Half of the time, headaches will develop in the course of non-strenuous activity, often during sleep. Headaches vary in intensity, location, duration, and response to treatment, thereby adding to the clinical challenge of recognizing that a subarachnoid hemorrhage has occurred. The diagnostic challenge is further compounded by the diversity of signs and symptoms (see **Table 1**). This complex and varied presentation often leads to misdiagnosis and delay of potentially lifesaving interventions. Thus, a proper response to someone complaining of the worst headache of his or her life is a trip to an emergency room, where appropriate diagnostic and treatment procedures can be initiated.

Table 1 Signs and Symptoms of Subarachnoid Hemorrhage

Low-grade fever	Nausea
Neck pain	Vomiting
Irritability	Ocular signs
Confusion	Seizures
Agitation	Severe headaches

20. I am a long-time migraine sufferer. Can you explain to me why my head hurts so much?

Migraine headaches
Neurological condition characterized by unilateral throbbing headaches, that are accompanied by nausea, vomiting, and hypersensitivity to light and sound. Migraines affect women much more frequently than men.

Migraine headaches are the most common group of severe primary headaches; approximately one in seven individuals will experience one in the course of their lifetime. Migraine attacks are spontaneous, characterized by unilateral throbbing headaches that are accompanied by nausea, vomiting, and hypersensitivity to light and sound. They are made worse by movement. Most of the time, migraines are preceded by an "aura," which is a warning phenomenon based on a spreading wave of increased cortical brain activity, followed by a period of diminished activity. Typical manifestations of an aura include visual disturbances (scintillating moving lights), tunnel vision, vertigo, tingling, numbness, hypersensitivity to touch, temporary loss of speech, odd scents, and facial movements.

The causes of migraine headaches are still a mystery.

The causes of migraine headaches are still a mystery. Most likely there is not a single triggering event, but rather an interaction of genetic vulnerabilities with stress, inflammation, and neural and vascular factors. Evidence suggests that meningeal pain receptors become sensitized by a variety of different events, including mechanical, chemical, or heat stimuli. Continuous exposure to these stimuli induces a relatively enduring functional change in the pain receptors. Chemicals released in response to pain stimuli can also cause dilatation of blood vessels. Subsequent fluid leakage into the tissue prompts the release of more inflammatory molecules, which further aggravates the pain, establishing a vicious cycle. The same sensory nerves that project to the meninges and the blood vessels in the brain also supply the face and the area around the eye, which may be a likely explanation for the "referred" symptoms that are so common during migraines. Central sensitization, accompanied by synaptic changes in pain-processing brain areas and inadequate pain inhibition, may be responsible for the sustained vulnerability toward migraines. Insufficient serotonin-related signaling has also been implicated in the origin of migraines. Because serotonin has a role in regulating the stress response, blood vessel tone, and emotional and pain modulation, its dysfunction is a likely contributing factor.

21. I have been experiencing excruciating headaches for several years. My doctor has recently diagnosed me with cluster headaches. What are they, and why does my head hurt so much?

Cluster headaches are characterized by clearly delineated pain attacks in the areas around the eye socket and forehead. Cluster headaches tend to be associated with a dysfunction of autonomic nerves, and symptoms can include drooping eyelids, pupil constriction (narrowing of pupils), teary eyes, runny nose, and sweating. Sometimes the pain will spread toward the cheek, lower jaw, and neck. Attacks usually come in clusters (hence the name) separated by symptom-free weeks or even years. Less than 10% of patients have a chronic form of the disorder without complete relief. Women are mostly spared from cluster headaches; up to 85% of the sufferers are male. Several factors have been implicated

Cluster headaches
Characterized by clearly delineated pain attacks in the innervation area of the first branch of the trigeminal nerve impacting the areas around the eye socket and forehead.

Introduction to Pain and Pain Disorders

in the origination of cluster headaches. Lack of balance between sympathetic signaling (involving norepinephrine) and parasympathetic activity (mediated by acetylcholine) may cause the release of inflammatory chemicals. These substances promote dilatation of blood vessels, as demonstrated by ultrasound studies showing an increased blood flow in the brain during cluster headache attacks. Additionally, the regulation of daily biorhythms may be compromised in patients with cluster headaches, suggesting an explanation for the unusual time pattern of the attacks.

22. I have suffered from severe neck pain radiating into my shoulder and arm for a couple of weeks. My doctor said that I will need a workup for cervical radiculopathy. What is that?

Cervical radiculopathy

Neuropathic pain due to injury of the cervical nerve roots, most often caused by compression. Commonly manifests as pain in the neck and one arm, and is associated with weakness and a loss of sensation in the area affected by nerve-root distribution.

Cervical radiculopathy—compression of the nerve root in the neck—commonly manifests as pain in the neck and one arm and is associated with weakness and a loss of sensation in the affected area. The most common cause of cervical radiculopathy is the compression of the cervical nerve due to changes in shape of one of the cervical discs (neck spine) or degenerative processes affecting the cervical (neck) vertebrae. Unlike the situation in the lumbar spine, herniated nucleus pulposus (a jelly-like substance in the middle of the spine disc) is rarely the cause of radiculopathy. Likewise, tumors, circulatory problems, and inflammation only occasionally cause this condition. Most often, inflammatory chemicals are released into the injured area by any of a variety of causes. Hypoxia—lack of oxygen due to inadequate blood supply—and inflammation of the nerve root and dorsal ganglia further aggravate the impact of the cord compression that most commonly causes this condition. An MRI (magnetic resonance imaging) study can be a very helpful diagnostic tool in the evaluation of radiculopathy. If disc herniation, also known as a "slipped disc," which is a tear in the fibrous ring encasing the nuclus pulposus and its subsequent protrusion, is the cause of radiculopathy, symptomatic relief coincides with radiologic evidence of retraction of the hernia.

23. Why do patients with multiple sclerosis experience so much pain?

Multiple sclerosis (MS) is an immune-mediated neurological disorder that typically follows a relapsing-remitting course. The disease typically starts with sensory disturbances, double vision, limb weakness, clumsiness, gait disturbance, fatigue, and bladder and bowel problems. Eventually, thought and emotional problems, including affective lability, vertigo, pain, and widespread loss of strength and sensation, may develop.

Pain is a prominent symptom in 30% to 85% of MS patients. Severity of this pain ranges from moderate to excruciating. Sadly, only a few patients experience mild pain. Pain in MS has multiple causes. Optic neuritis (inflammation of the optic nerve), painful spasms, central nervous system lesions, trigeminal neuralgia, musculoskeletal back pain, and headache are some of the main sources of MS pain. As in all medical and psychiatric conditions, the presence of pain in MS substantially increases the disease burden and negatively impacts the quality of the patient's life.

24. What is the cause of low back pain?

Epidemiologic studies suggest that approximately two-thirds of adults experience back pain at some point in their lives. **Low back pain (LBP)** is also one of the most frequent reasons people seek medical attention,

Multiple sclerosis (MS)

An immune-mediated neurological disorder that typically follows a relapsing-remitting course.

Low back pain (LBP)

Pain that originates from spinal ligaments, facet joints, the periosteum, paravertebral muscles, fascia, and compressed spinal nerve roots. Most commonly, the pain is of musculoskeletal origin related to the degeneration of facet joints and intervertebral disks.

31

second only to respiratory illness. Fortunately, episodes of back pain most often are short lived and resolve spontaneously. Low back pain affects women and men with equal frequency, and most cases develop in individuals between the ages of 30 to 50 years. It is the leading cause of disability in people under the age of 45.

Low back pain can develop from any of several causes. Whatever the cause, most of the pain originates from spinal ligaments, facet joints, the connective tissue enveloping the bones, paravertebral muscles and fascia, and compressed spinal nerve roots. Most commonly, the pain is of musculoskeletal origin, related to the degeneration of facet joints and intervertebral disks. Another, somewhat less frequent cause of back pain is **spinal stenosis**. This condition is caused by narrowing of the central spinal canal or lateral recesses, most often due to age-related hypertrophy (enlargement) of joint facets or thickening of ligaments, either of which cause compression of the spinal cord and the nerves. Other reasons for lower back pain include fracture caused by osteoporosis or trauma, congenital disease, disk disruption, tumors, infections, and inflammatory disease.

Spinal stenosis

Caused by narrowing of the central spinal canal or lateral recesses, most often due to age-related hypertrophy of joint facets or thickening of ligamentum flavum, either of which cause compression of the spinal cord and the nerves.

Unfortunately, in most individuals the precise cause of their LBP remains unknown. Consistent with this, about 85% of patients are classified as having "nonspecific low back pain." Vague terms like degeneration, strain, and sprain are used to explain the cause of pain when more specific causes are not readily identifiable. In reality, there is virtually no structural abnormality to explain the cause of pain in most people with LBP. Indeed, the relationship between clinical symptoms and imaging findings is weak at best. Fortunately, 90% of LBP episodes are acute and resolve within 3 months, and usually within 2 weeks. Only 10% of people with acute back pain go on to develop chronic LBP. Unfortunately, 40% of patients with short-term LBP will suffer a recurrence within 6 months. An exception to this pattern may be spinal stenosis, which tends to remain stable, with only a small percentage of patients experiencing improvement or worsening over time.

Chronic back pain can be associated with peripheral and central sensitization. When sensitization develops, pain receptive fibers have greater sensitivity, while spinal nerve cells facilitate transmission of pain signals to brain centers involved in pain perception and processing. Lasting structural changes in these pain-processing brain areas have also been described in the context of chronic back pain. Interestingly, one of the affected areas is a brain region involved in working memory, concentration, and decision-making. One might wonder if these structural brain changes underlie the difficulty with memory, attention, and problem solving that is so often reported by our patients with chronic LBP. These enduring functional and structural changes in the pain-processing areas may explain why the pain does not stop even in the absence of a clear cause. It is as if the brain has "learned" to experience exaggerated pain, and this learning has "rewired" the brain.

25. How does one diagnose low back pain?

A diagnosis of low back pain (LBP) starts with a focused medical history. Risk factors for LBP include an age older than 50 years, a history of cancer or unexplained weight loss (pain related to malignancy), intravenous drug use or chronic infections, nighttime pain (malignant pain and inflammatory pain not relieved by rest), and systemic steroids (osteoporosis). Inflammatory arthritis of the hips and knee may point to **spondylitis** (inflammation of the vertebra). Neurological deficits

Spondylitis

Inflamed or degenerated joints between different vertebrae in the spine. Symptoms include leg pain after walking, tingling, and numbness.

such as leg pain after walking, tingling, and numbness are often associated with this condition. If pain intensifies with sneezing and coughing, this may point to disk herniation as a cause of the back pain. Compression of the cauda equina (the lowest portion of the spinal cord; see **Figure 9**) may produce problems with the bladder and bowels and may impair sexual function. Cauda equina compression is usually caused by a tumor or midline herniation. Patients with cauda equina compression are also likely to complain of numbness in the "saddle area." Information about depression, anxiety, work, family, and financial stress can also be helpful. Involvement with litigation or pursuit of disability may at times be associated with vague, difficult to interpret symptoms.

A physical exam can sometimes provide crucial information. Fever and vertebral tenderness can be suggestive

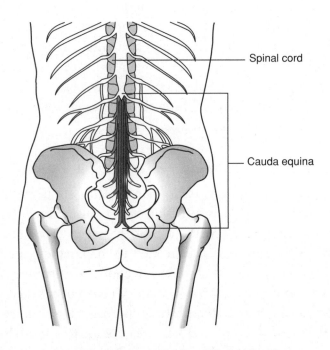

Spinal cord

Cauda equina

Figure 9   Cauda equina: The lowest portion of the spinal cord.

of inflammation. Ankylosing spondylitis, which is chronic inflammatory arthritis of the spine, is likely to be associated with limited chest expansion. An elevation of less than 60% on a straight leg-raising test can be indicative of nerve-root compression or irritation. In this case, a positive test will reproduce the symptoms of sciatica. Evaluation of motor strength and sensation will provide useful information about possible disk herniation and ensuing neurological problems.

Diagnostic imaging is not indicated for the 85% of the LBP sufferers who have the "nonspecific" variant. Overall, an MRI is the best procedure when radicular compression is due to a herniated disc, spinal stenosis (narrowing of spinal canal), tumor, systemic disease, or infection.

26. What is phantom limb pain?

As bizarre as it is, phantom limb pain is nothing new—in fact, it was first described in the mid-sixteenth century. For several hundred years it was considered a form of insanity or a proof of the existence of the soul. The term *phantom limb phenomenon* refers to the sense that a part of the body that has been amputated is still present. **Phantom limb pain (PLP)** tends to occur most often at the far end of the missing limb, such as in the hands or feet. For example, if the lower limb has been amputated, pain will be experienced in the area where the toes, heel, ankle, and instep were. Phantom limb pain is typically characterized by intermittent burning, cramping, stinging, throbbing, tearing, or piercing pain. Most often PLP will develop in days or weeks after amputation, but on rare occasions it can start several months later. Because PLP has a relatively stable early course, 60% to 70% of amputees who develop PLP will continue to report this strange pain a year later.

Phantom limb pain (PLP)

Localized predominantly in the distal part of the missing limb. For example, if the lower limb has been amputated, pain will be experienced in the area where the toes, heel, ankle, and instep were, even though they are no longer attached to the person's body.

Introduction to Pain and Pain Disorders

Fortunately, however, the majority of PLP sufferers experience some relief with the passage of time.

Both the peripheral and central nervous system appear to contribute to the development of PLP, although its exact cause remains unknown. Like many other forms of pain, it may be related to central sensitization in which the central nervous system becomes inappropriately sensitive to signals from the body or even begins to perceive painful sensations for which there is no bodily cause. Studies have shown that when pain fibers from the periphery are cut (such as happens with amputation) dorsal horn neurons in the spinal cord that process pain signals from the periphery of the body begin to fire more often in response to less and less stimulation. Nerve fibers also begin to grow in incorrect ways, leading to "crazy wiring" that confuses touch with pain.

In addition to nerves getting "crossed" in the spinal cord, there is evidence that PLP is also associated with altered function and structure of the brain. For example, studies have shown that direct stimulation of an area of the brain called the thalamus can reproduce the symptoms of PLP even in the absence of an amputation. More and more studies also suggest that PLP is perpetuated by changes in the organization of cortical brain regions, especially in somatosensory and motor areas responsible for sensation and movement. Neuroimaging studies show that shifts in how the severed limb is represented in the brain correlate with the incidence and severity of PLP. A leading hypothesis is that motor areas of the brain send out a continuous outflow of neural activity from areas that correspond to the missing limb. Because the limb is missing, there is no regulatory sensory feedback or—worse yet—there is scrambled feedback. This lack of feedback may promote PLP over time.

27. Two months ago my leg was injured in a motor vehicle accident. Although my doctors told me that there was no nerve injury and my leg looks completely healed, it is still red and swollen, and the skin is sweaty. Sometimes it is just tender, but on other occasions it is outright painful. What is wrong with me?

Based on your description, a condition called **Complex Regional Pain Syndrome (CRPS)** is the most likely cause of your pain. CRPS is a combined inflammatory and neuropathic pain disorder that usually develops after a limb injury. This condition is characterized by excessive pain (hyperalgesia); tenderness to touch (allodynia); tingling and numbness; sweaty, flushed skin of abnormal temperature; and impairment of motion in the affected area. The causes of CRPS have not been completely discovered, but it appears that peripheral and central nervous system factors combine to generate the symptoms of CRPS. In the periphery of the body, CRPS has been associated with nerve sensitization, an increase in inflammatory molecules called cytokines in the skin, and more general inflammation that is caused by inappropriate nerve activity. Blood vessel walls often function abnormally in this condition, which robs the affected area of needed oxygen.

Contributions from the central nervous system are equally well substantiated. Changes in central motor pathways result in muscle weakness, tremors, and abnormal muscle tone in the affected area of the body. Altered somatosensory cortical responses to touch and changes in cortical representation of the affected areas often develop. Structural brain scans show that CRPS is associated with reduced volume in a number of brain

Complex Regional Pain Syndrome (CRPS)

A combined inflammatory and neuropathic pain disorder, which usually develops after a limb injury. This condition is characterized by excessive pain (hyperalgesia); tenderness to touch (allodynia); tingling and numbness; sweaty; flushed skin of abnormal temperature; and impairment of motion.

regions that are also important for emotions and respond-ing to stress. These areas include the insula, ventrome-dial prefrontal cortex, and right nucleus accumbens. Studies have also found that patients with CRPS have pathological changes in how cortical and subcortical brain areas are connected to each other. The more widespread these changes, the more severe and long-standing the pain. Fortunately, imaging evidence also suggests that successful treatment may reverse these brain changes and the symptoms they cause.

28. What is carpal tunnel syndrome?

**Carpal tunnel
syndrome (CTS)**

Painful condition caused by compres-sion of a major nerve passing through a narrow space defined by carpal bones, ten-dons, and soft tissue. Tissue swelling will compress the nerve, causing tingling, burning, and numb-ness impacting the palmar side of the thumb, index finger, middle finger, and half of the ring finger.

Carpal tunnel syndrome (CTS) is a common pain syn-drome associated with significant disability. More than 2.5 million U.S. medical office visits annually are related to finger, hand, and wrist problems that qualify for a diagnosis of CTS. Despite its high prevalence, however, experts are not in full agreement about what causes CTS. While many consider it to be a specific type of neuropathic pain, others think that it may be better classified as pain of mixed origin given the important role that inflammation plays in its development.

The carpal tunnel is located at the base of the palm (see **Figure 10**). It is bounded on three sides by carpal bones, and on the fourth side it is "covered" by the transverse carpal ligament. The median nerve and nine flexor tendons traverse the carpal tunnel. Any increase in the pressure within the carpal tunnel can lead to compression and ischemia of median nerve producing pain and a tingling sensation within its area of distri-bution. Pressure on the tunnel area can be generated by repetitive, forceful wrist movements. When the compression is repeated over time, the median nerve may lose its myelin covering, which can lead to loss of function and feelings of pain. In addition to overuse,

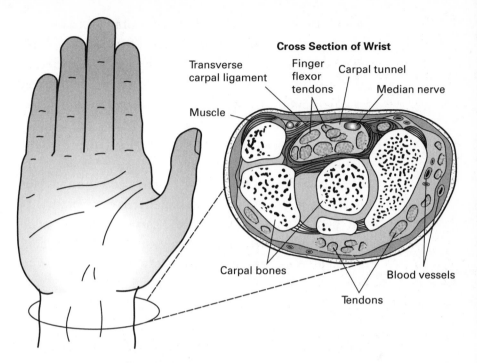

Figure 10   The carpal tunnel is located at the base of the palm.

other conditions can increase the risk for CTS, including infections, diabetes, hypothyroidism, pregnancy, and use of steroids or estrogens. Some people are born with physical abnormalities of the carpal tunnel, which also increases the risk of CTS.

CTS usually begins with pain, tingling, burning, or numbness on the palm side of the thumb, as well as the index and middle finger and half of the ring finger. These symptoms are initially most common in the late afternoon and nighttime, but eventually become continuous throughout the day. Those with a moderate/severe form of this condition additionally will have weakness in the affected hand. This can lead to an inability to grip objects with the hand, which can be a source of great frustration.

If you are experiencing these types of symptoms, it is important that you see your doctor. He or she will likely do a physical exam to check for the most classic finding of CTS, which is a loss of ability to recognize whether you are being touched in one or two places simultaneously in the affected area. Your doctor may also press on the carpal tunnel area of your wrist or may inflate a blood pressure cuff over that arm to see whether the inflation produces feelings of tingling and numbness in the areas of your arm and hand that are innervated by the median nerve trapped in the carpal tunnel. In addition to these more basic exams, your doctor may order a test called a nerve conduction study to see if signals are being disrupted or slowed in the median nerve.

29. I have heard of carpal tunnel, but my friend mentioned that he is suffering from tarsal tunnel syndrome. What is that?

Tarsal tunnel syndrome (TTS)

A painful neuropathic condition caused by compression of the posterior tibial nerve in the tarsal tunnel, which is a part of the foot where ligaments form a space (a tunnel) through which this nerve travels. When the tunnel is narrowed, the nerve is compressed, causing pain.

Tarsal tunnel syndrome (TTS) is a painful neuropathic condition caused by compression of the posterior tibial nerve in the tarsal tunnel. More simply, it is very much like carpal tunnel syndrome, but in the foot instead of the hand. The tarsal tunnel is a narrow space located on the inner side of the ankle (see **Figure 11**). The tunnel is formed by a bone called the medial malleolus, bony structures of the ankle, and ligaments that attach the flexor leg muscles to leg bones. The tibial nerve and artery, as well as the tendons of flexor muscles, pass through this tarsal tunnel and thus are at risk for damage should the tunnel itself sustain damage. As with the hand, repetitive overuse of the leg flexor muscles (most common in athletes), prolonged standing or walking, or pregnancy are all capable of causing swelling in the tarsal tunnel, which then can compress the tibial nerve. Other less common causes of

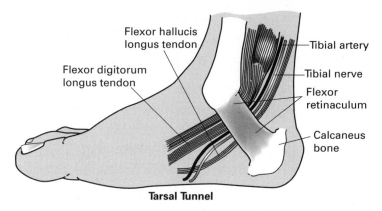

Tarsal Tunnel

Figure 11 **The tarsal tunnel is a narrow space located on the inner side of the ankle.**

TTS include cysts, bone spurs, and trauma to the area. Occasionally people with lower back pain can develop linked inflammation in the tarsal tunnel, which can also produce TTS. Pain in this condition is caused by a combination of nerve compression, inflammation, and lack of oxygen to the area.

People with TTS often complain of pain radiating along the inner side of the foot to the big toe and the first three toes. The pain is described as burning or stinging and is often accompanied by tingling, "hot and cold" sensations and numbness. Reports of swelling and numbness involving the heel and sole of the affected foot are less frequent. The pain is made worse by standing and prolonged activity and is relieved with rest. A good history and examination are usually sufficient for diagnosis. Tindel's sign, elicited by tapping on the tarsal tunnel area, typically causes spreading tingling and discomfort in the affected area. Electrophysiological studies and MRI can provide additional diagnostic information.

30. I wake up every morning with a pain in the bottom of my foot. My doctor told me that I have plantar fasciitis. What is that?

Plantar fasciitis is a chronic pain disorder affecting close to 2 million Americans. Most often one experiences a sharp stabbing pain in the heel of the foot upon taking the first few steps after awakening. The pain usually affects only one foot. Plantar fasciitis can also be triggered by standing or getting up after sitting for a long time. Plantar fasciitis pain gradually eases with resumption of activity and tends to get worse toward evening. It is particularly common in runners, overweight individuals, and pregnant women. This painful condition is more often diagnosed in the elderly and individuals with extensive work-related weight bearing, especially when done wearing shoes with little arch support. If plantar fasciitis persists without treatment it can lead to degenerative changes in the foot.

The plantar fascia is a thick band of connective tissue that supports the bones at the bottom of the foot. Although the exact causes are not known, plantar fasciitis occurs when this tissue becomes inflamed or begins to break down. If your doctor suspects plantar fasciitis, he or she will probably conduct a test for it that involves bending your toes up toward your shin. If you have plantar fasciitis this will cause a very sharp pain. In addition to this very simple test, your doctor may order more "high-tech" studies if there is any reason to worry that you might have another cause for your symptoms.

31. What is post–herpetic neuralgia?

Post-herpetic neuralgia (PHN) is a debilitating, painful condition that develops following a flare-up of the herpes zoster virus (known as "shingles"). Unfortunately, the risk of developing PHN increases with age.

The time frame for the onset of PHN pain extends from rash resolution up to 3 months after rash onset. The pain that accompanies PHN can be long-standing: about 1 in 10 patients report experiencing significant pain 6 months after their herpes zoster exacerbation. Most often the pain comes and goes, is not related to external triggers, and paradoxically affects skin areas that lack normal sensitivity. PHN pain is usually described as burning, throbbing, and aching. Typically, these pain attacks are short-lived and do not interfere with sleep. Sometimes patients with PHN will experience markedly increased pain responses, even in response to generally non-painful stimuli such as light touch on the skin. Painful areas in PHN can also be associated with itching and tingling sensations.

Although the exact causes of PHN are not known, a leading theory is that the symptoms are caused by viral damage to sensory nerves. Consistent with this, patients who receive antiviral therapy during herpes zoster virus exacerbations are less likely to experience burning PHN pain afterward.

32. What is diabetic neuropathy?

Diabetic neuropathy (often abbreviated as "**DNP**" for diabetic neuropathic pain) is a common complication of both type I and type II diabetes. In fact, between 15% and 30% of diabetic patients will go on to develop DNP, which explains why DNP affects approximately 21 million Americans. Unfortunately, maintaining good control of one's blood sugar does not appear to reduce the risk of developing DNP.

Patients commonly describe pain of DNP as sharp, stinging, burning, or aching, or like little electrical shocks. In addition to pain, DNP is typically characterized by

Diabetic neuropathy (DNP)

Condition caused by injury to the nerves, most likely due to microvascular disease. Small blood vessels supplying nerves are occluded due to diabetes and can no longer fulfill their role.

numbness and tingling; loss of sensation to temperature, pressure, or pain is also common. Diabetic neuropathy most often affects the hands and feet (see **Figure 12**). As the condition advances, affected limbs may lose normal reflexes. Patients with severe DNP

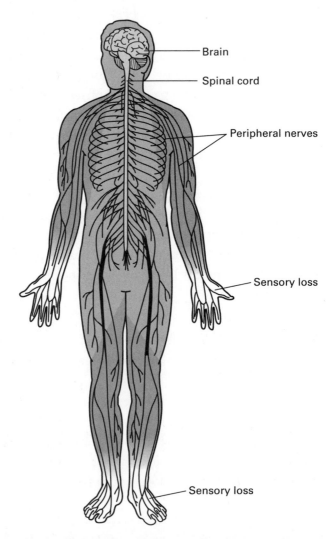

Figure 12   DNP most often affects the hands and feet ("the glove and stocking distribution"). As the condition advances, affected limbs may lose normal reflexes.

Introduction to Pain and Pain Disorders

eventually may become unable to walk. Sometimes DNP patients will experience pain upon light touch, which can make something as slight as bedsheets touching the skin unbearable. This and many other symptoms occur more often at night, which helps explain why DNP is so often associated with sleep disruption. This can start a vicious cycle, because sleep disturbance itself can increase pain sensations.

A good patient history and an examination that includes careful mapping and exploration of all pain and pain-related sensations are essential for correctly diagnosing DNP. Testing pain sensitivity (pin prick, two point discrimination), response to pressure, temperature (tubes of hot and cold water), vibration (tuning fork), muscular reflexes, and muscle strength are particularly relevant parts of the neurological examination of DNP patients (**Table 2**). Serial chemistry evaluating hemoglobin A1C can be a helpful measure of long-term glycemic control and renal function measures provide information regarding medication clearance issues. Nerve conduction studies are often helpful in providing information reflective of nerve demyelination and damage. However, while useful for diagnosing the condition, none of these studies correlate well with the symptomatic burden in DNP.

Table 2   Evaluation and Diagnosis of Diabetic Neuropathy

Pain sensitivity-pin prick	Response to pressure
Sensitivity to temperature	Vibration sensitivity (tuning fork)
Muscular reflexes	Muscle strength
Serial evaluation of hemoglobin A1C	Nerve conduction studies

33. How does diabetes cause neuropathy?

Many factors are known to increase the risk for diabetic neuropathy (DNP), but the primary abnormality for this condition appears to lie within very small blood vessels known as the microvasculature. Diabetic neuropathy appears to develop as a result of the walls of very small blood vessels becoming thicker to the point that the vessels become plugged. When this happens, blood flow stops and nearby nerves become starved for oxygen and important nutrients they need to survive. As these nerves become compromised they further contribute to the problem by causing a condition known as arterio-venous shunting, in which blood flows directly from larger arterioles into the veins, entirely skipping the small vessels that supply nerves and other tissues. Given these findings, it comes as no surprise that increasing blood flow in small vessels improves neuropathic pain symptoms in affected areas.

When nerves and other tissues don't get enough oxygen, they begin to release inflammatory chemicals, which strongly activate pain-sensing nerves.

When nerves and other tissues don't get enough oxygen, they begin to release inflammatory chemicals, which strongly activate pain-sensing nerves. This activation makes pain pathways in the spinal cord and brain increasingly sensitive to pain signals, sometimes becoming so sensitized that they perceive pain when no signals are coming from the body. This process is called central sensitization, and it is believed to underlie many chronic pain conditions. When pain pathways become sensitized, this seems, over time, to cause changes in the structure of areas of the brain that are important for recognizing and reacting to pain signals from the body. These changes appear to reflect damage to these areas. Normally these areas deep in the brain play an important role in what is known as the "descending inhibitory pain pathway." This pathway allows the brain to turn down the intensity of pain sensations. When damaged, these brain areas become less able to turn down the intensity of these pain signals, which is recognized as an important process in many chronic pain conditions. The downward inhibitory pain pathway utilizes a number of signaling molecules, including opioids, serotonin, and norepinephrine, all of which have been targeted by various classes of pain control medications.

34. Why do people with irritable bowel syndrome experience so much pain?

Although defined by the gastrointestinal symptoms reflected in its name, **irritable bowel syndrome (IBS)** also is commonly associated with prominent pain symptoms. In this regard, other chronic painful conditions such as interstitial cystitis, chronic pelvic pain, dyspareunia (pain during intercourse), dysmenorrhea (painful menstruation), endometriosis, migraine headaches, back pain, TMJ, fibromyalgia, and chronic fatigue often accompany IBS. Emotional pain is also quite common, given that psychiatric disorders have been reported in 94% of IBS patients. Approximately 12% of Americans suffer from IBS, and it is the reason for 20% to 50% of referrals to gastroenterologists. Seventy percent of IBS patients are women. Irritable bowel syndrome has been classified into three subtypes: (A) predominantly painful, (B) primarily constipation-related, and (C) diarrhea-related.

Patients with IBS will often complain of chronic, recurrent abdominal pain relieved by defecation, accompanied by disturbance of bowel habits, bloating, and discomfort. These symptoms are believed to be caused by several processes. IBS shares with other chronic pain conditions the pathology of sensitization in which nerve cells become overly responsive to signals and thus amplify pain sensations. IBS is also characterized by

Irritable bowel syndrome (IBS)

Chronic functional digestive disorder characterized by recurrent abdominal pain, relieved by defecation, and accompanied by disturbance of bowel habits, bloating, and discomfort in the absence of an identifiable organic cause.

"visceral hypersensitivity," which means that people with the condition complain of more pain than others in response to sensations in the gut. This has been shown experimentally by measuring the amount of pain felt when the gut is mechanically "puffed up." While nobody likes this feeling, patients with IBS complain of far more discomfort than people without the condition. This visceral hypersensitivity seems to be related to the fact that patients with IBS release more pain-promoting neurotransmitters in their gut than others. These responses promote inflammation in the nerves which makes them even more sensitive to pain signals over time. Thus, IBS is characterized by abnormalities that increase the amount of pain signal that gets to the brain. But as with all chronic pain conditions, the brain begins to function abnormally over time and loses its ability to suppress pain signals coming from the gut. As we have discussed in regard to other pain problems, the system by which the brain dampens down pain signaling is called the "descending inhibitory pathway." Medications like antidepressants that have been shown to help with IBS probably do so by restoring the activity in this pathway, allowing the brain (and the person!) to not constantly feel discomfort in response to even minor types of stimulation.

The gut is sometimes called the "second brain" because it has so many nerve cells. These nerve cells communicate back and forth with the brain. Research increasingly shows that how a person feels emotionally gets transmitted to the gut, and how the gut is functioning sends signals to the brain that affect how a person feels emotionally. Given this, it's no surprise that conditions like depression, anxiety, and chronic stress aggravate IBS symptoms. These conditions are associated with increased inflammation, and as we've already said, increased inflammation contributes to the development of IBS. So it makes sense that emotional distress can actually produce physical changes that promote IBS. Current thinking suggests that IBS can also be caused by problems in the gut itself, which of course makes sense. Some evidence suggests that infection of the gut by bacteria or protozoal organisms can set IBS in motion, as can a poorly functioning autonomic nervous system in the gut. Often these factors cluster together, making it impossible to pinpoint a specific cause for any given person's IBS symptoms.

35. My husband has been avoiding intercourse lately due to pain in his prostate. He saw a doctor who diagnosed it as prostatodynia. What is this, and is it curable?

Prostatodynia is a common urogenital pain disorder of unknown origin that typically occurs in men between the ages of 20 to 60 years. Patients suffering from prostatodynia often complain of pain on urination, urinary urgency followed by poor urinary flow, and pain in the pelvic floor. Patients with this condition will often also complain of more widespread pain affecting the groin, lower back, and suprapubic areas, as well as intense pain at the time of ejaculation.

If you are suffering with these symptoms, your doctor will first make sure that some other clearly identifiable factor is not causing your problem. Potential causes for these symptoms other than prostatodynia include infections of the prostate as well as allergic or autoimmune conditions affecting the prostate. Interestingly, despite the intensely painful symptoms, men with prostatodynia are usually normal on physical examination. However, high-tech urodynamic studies have identified more subtle abnormalities in the function of the urethral sphincter

Prostatodynia

A common urogenital pain disorder of unknown origin, typically occurring in men between the ages of 20 to 60 years. Patients suffering from prostatodynia often complain of pain during urination, urinary urgency followed by poor urinary flow, and pain in the pelvic floor.

in some patients with the condition. As with other chronic pain conditions, psychological factors appear to contribute to the development of prostatodynia, which is consistent with the fact that stress alters the activity of autonomic nerves that are important for prostate functioning. Psychological factors that have been implicated in the development of prostatodynia include anxiety, depression, relationship struggles, and a past history of unsatisfactory sexual functioning. Men with prostatodynia also often have symptoms of conditions such as fibromyalgia and chronic fatigue syndrome. Because these conditions are associated with changes in how the central nervous system processes pain, it is possible that subtle changes in the functioning and structure of the spinal cord may also contribute to prostatodynia.

Various forms of treatment including exercise, relaxation therapy, psychotherapy, biofeedback, and pharmacotherapy (anxiolytic and antidepressant medicines) have all been known to greatly ease the symptoms of prostatodynia.

36. I have always experienced pain with intercourse and when inserting a tampon. My gynecologist told me that I might be suffering from vulvodynia. What is that?

Vulvodynia

A chronic pain syndrome lasting at least 3 months manifested by vulvar (external female genitalia) discomfort, burning and/or stinging pain, irritation, and dyspareunia (painful or uncomfortable intercourse).

Vulvodynia (also known as the "burning vulva syndrome") is a chronic pain syndrome lasting at least 3 months that is characterized by vulvar discomfort, burning and stinging pain, irritation, and dyspareunia (painful intercourse). Women have also described pain during insertion of tampons or a speculum. The onset of this pain can vary widely, from very sudden to very gradual. Sometimes the pain is localized to the genital area. In other cases it involves the entire pelvic area and can even spread up the back. Vulvodynia is often aggravated by walking, running, exercise, horseback riding, bicycling, urination, and wearing tight-fitting clothes. Although its exact prevalence isn't known, vulvodynia appears to be fairly common. Some studies suggest that 15% of women seen in gynecology offices suffer from the condition.

The onset of vulvodynia pain has been linked to vaginal infection, surgery in the vulvo-vaginal area, sexual trauma, and changes in pattern of sexual activity. A number of studies suggest that relationship factors can strongly influence the condition. Ambivalent relationships seem to contribute to vulvodynia, and connected to this, sexual intercourse prior to—or without—adequate arousal and lubrication may also contribute to the condition. Consistent with a role for stress in pain development, women with vulvodynia are at increased risk for depression, anxiety, chronic stress, and other types of physical symptoms for which a clear-cut medical cause cannot be found. Other factors thought to increase the risk for vulvodynia include infections, a poor diet, and genes that promote autoimmunity.

As with many chronic pain conditions, the exact cause of vulvodynia is unknown, but evidence increasingly suggests a process known as sensitization. If you've read through the preceding questions you'll know that this describes a pathological process whereby changes occur in nerves and the brain regions to which they connect to make them increasingly sensitive to pain signals. When full-blown, peripheral and central sensitization can lead to states in which severe pain is perceived by the brain in the absence of any significant source in the body for the pain. One of the reasons researchers think that vulvodynia develops as a result of sensitization is that, like other disorders with this feature, it is often associated with allodynia (when even light touch on the skin hurts), hyperalgesia (when pain sensations are markedly increased), and sensations of tingling.

If you are suffering with vulvodynia symptoms, don't be surprised if you go to the doctor and he or she tells you that your physical exam is normal. This is typical. Because the condition does not usually have diagnostic physical or laboratory findings, it is what is called a "diagnosis of exclusion," meaning that women are only considered to have vulvodynia when other known diseases that could cause the symptoms have been ruled out.

37. What are the causes of chronic rectal pain?

Chronic rectal pain can be divided into two types that have different causes and usually different outcomes. The first type of rectal pain is called **proctodynia**, and it is characterized by constant rectal pain. The second type is called **proctalgia fugax**, and it is characterized by rapid bouts of pain that come and go. Let's talk about proctodynia first. This type of chronic rectal pain is usually due to a disease process that is directly affecting the rectum, such as a painful anal fissure. Every once in a while chronic rectal pain comes not from the rectum itself but from a nearby organ. This type of pain is called "referred pain" because the source of pain is one place, but the sensation of the pain is felt someplace else. In the case of proctodynia, the source of pain can sometimes be in the urinary tract or even the lower spine. People with these conditions often also will have symptoms of vulvodynia if they are women or prostodynia if they are men. A number of clear-cut diseases can also cause proctodynia. For example, chronic rectal pain can be experienced in people with a bulging back disc, or with a tumor that is pushing against the nerves of the lowest part of the spinal cord. When no clear-cut

Proctodynia

Characterized by constant pain in the rectal/anal area of the body.

Proctalgia fugax

Characterized by fleeting, paroxysmal pain of the rectal/anus.

cause is found, patients will sometimes be found to have a poorly functioning external anal sphincter. When chronic rectal pain comes from this type of more subtle functional abnormality, psychological factors (e.g., anxiety, depression, life stress) are often found to be present in the individual.

The second type of chronic rectal pain, proctalgia fugax, has been described in the medical literature for more than a century. It is characterized by sudden, at times excruciating, brief attacks of pain in the area of the anus. These attacks tend to occur irregularly. In some individuals they last for weeks, while in others they persist for years. Although the exact cause of this condition is not known, most of the research done to date suggests that these symptoms most likely arise from dysfunction of the smooth muscles that ring the gastrointestinal tract and help to push food and waste material along for removal from the body. Another potential cause of proctalgia fugax may be changes in the blood vessels that supply the anus, resulting in vasospasm, during which the blood vessels clamp down and prevent needed oxygen and nutrients from reaching the anal area.

If you have either of these painful conditions, make sure your doctor does a careful rectal exam to rule out an obvious cause like a tumor. But be prepared for your exam to be normal—especially if you've had your symptoms for a long time. This is quite common in patients with chronic rectal pain.

38. What can you tell me about the cause of pain associated with rheumatoid arthritis?

Rheumatoid arthritis (RA) is an autoimmune disorder characterized by chronic inflammation in many joints of

Rheumatoid arthritis (RA)

An autoimmune disorder (when "confused" immune system turns against our own tissue, "mistaking" it for a foreign substance) characterized by chronic inflammation of multiple joints, associated with destruction of cartilage and adjoining bony structures.

the body that often leads to destruction of the cartilage and bony structures of which joints are made. The most common symptoms of RA are pain and stiffness in the affected joints. Over time many people with RA will show clear X-ray evidence of damage to their joints, but interestingly the amount of pain and joint damage patients experience do not usually go hand in hand.

This mismatch between the intensity of pain a patient feels and findings of joint damage on X-ray is particularly common early in the disease course. Unfortunately, as the disease progresses, the arthritis pain usually gets worse, so that over time people become more vulnerable to feeling pain in response to lower levels of provocation. By now the reader should recognize this as the kind of peripheral and/or central pain sensitization that is believed to underlie many chronic pain conditions. Sensitization of the central nervous system in RA likely explains why many patients begin to feel pain that extends beyond the affected joints, why psychological stress worsens the pain, and why many people with RA will also meet criteria for fibromyalgia—a widespread pain condition in which central sensitization is believed to play a primary role.

Susan, a 50-year-old female with RA, really highlights many points we've made in this section about how the disease changes over time as a result of nervous system sensitization:

When I was first diagnosed with rheumatoid arthritis 16 years ago, I was most bothered by swelling, soreness, and stiffness in my knees and ankles. Certainly the pain limited my life; I wasn't able to do many of the things that I used to enjoy such as playing sports and hiking, but I thought that I could control the pain by protecting my joints, getting enough rest, and doing non-impact exercises. Over the years, however, the pain has changed. The swelling and stiffness has not gone away, but this is not the most painful part of the experience any more. The most distressing pain is less specific. My entire body aches, it hurts to be touched, and I am sometimes reluctant to even put my feet on the floor for fear of the pressure that I will feel against my soles. I also feel it in the form of deep exhaustion; I am so tired that it is difficult to fulfill my daily responsibilities, but I'm in so much pain that I can't sleep. It makes me irritable, moody, and sad. It affects my relationships because I don't want to be touched and I don't want to interact. During a flare-up I just want to curl up in a ball and be left alone.

39. What is the role of depression in rheumatoid arthritis pain?

Depression often precedes the onset of RA, and many people who first develop RA will later go on to suffer with depression. Thus each condition appears to be a risk factor for the other. Not only are depression and RA risk factors for each other, but in patients with RA, intensity of depression is associated with intensity of arthritic pain, which means that the more depressed an RA patient is, the more intense his or her pain is likely to be, but also that the worse the pain is, the worse the depression is likely to be.

This close relationship between RA and depression may reflect more than just the fact that stress makes you hurt and that hurting makes you unhappy. Indeed, many studies now show that depression and RA share a number of abnormalities in the body and brain that may help explain why the two conditions so often occur together.

Both depression and RA are associated with a number of interconnected abnormalities in bodily systems that

Many studies now show that depression and RA share a number of abnormalities in the body and brain that may help explain why the two conditions so often occur together.

evolved to deal with stress and infection. Two primary systems connect the brain with the body and work to provide energy to deal with acute danger. These systems are called the hypothalamic-pituitary-adrenal (HPA) axis and the autonomic nervous system. The autonomic nervous system, in turn, has two branches: the sympathetic, which helps drive stress responses, and the parasympathetic, which helps promote relaxation and bodily restoration. In general, both depression and RA are associated with increased activity of the sympathetic system and reduced activity of the parasympathetic system. In terms of the HPA axis, many patients with RA and/or depression show an abnormal resistance to the primary HPA axis hormone cortisol. Because cortisol is highly anti-inflammatory, the fact that both RA and depression are syndromes of cortisol resistance may be one of the factors that promote increased inflammation in both illnesses. Similarly, although it is complicated, it appears that heightened sympathetic activity generally promotes inflammation, whereas parasympathetic activity, which is reduced in RA and depression, is strongly anti-inflammatory.

Many brain areas that register and respond to physical pain in the body are also activated by emotionally painful states such as anxiety and depression. Not surprisingly, therefore, a number of studies find that RA and depression tend to be associated with similar abnormalities in a number of brain regions, especially the amydgala, hippocampus, anterior cingulate cortex, and medial prefrontal cortex. Scientists increasingly suspect that these altered patterns of brain activity may also play a big role in the **comorbidity** between depression and RA.

Comorbidity

An accompanying condition to a previous illness.

Brian, a 40-year-old male, tells a story that really brings home the close physiological connections in brain and body between physical and emotional pain:

Before I was diagnosed with depression I was seen by multiple doctors for a wide variety of painful symptoms. I had frequent headaches, neck pain, joint pain, and stomach pain. I was exhausted; I slept every chance I could get and still felt tired. I was sent to specialist after specialist and was treated for migraines and irritable bowel syndrome. When these treatments failed, I had an MRI and neurological tests to determine the source of my pain. Eventually, I was tested for everything from fibromyalgia to lupus. When all the tests came back negative I could tell that my doctors were losing patience with me. I suspected that they thought that I was a hypochondriac. I started to wonder about this myself. Could this pain be all in my imagination? Did I just want attention? It wasn't until I saw a therapist for other reasons that it became clear that I have a mood disorder. The treatment for this was the first thing that made a dent in my pain. Now I go to therapy, take medications for my depression, control my stress, eat correctly, and exercise. Although my pain has not disappeared, it is now manageable—I ache less, sleep less, and enjoy life more.

40. What is the origin of pain in osteoarthritis?

Osteoarthritis (OA) is the most common cause of pain in individuals older than 40 years of age, and in general the incidence of OA increases with age. A number of physical changes occur in the joints of patients with OA, all of which contribute to the development of pain in the condition. First, wear and tear on joints over time leads to bone and cartilage damage. This damage promotes an inflammatory response in affected joints, which then leads to a thickening of the joint capsule and the formation of new bone at inappropriate places in the joint. This causes the joint to further degenerate and fail, leading to inflammation that spreads to the syn-

Osteoarthritis (OA)
A painful degenerative condition of the joints, particularly affecting us with increasing age.

ovial membranes that encase the entire joint. In advanced OA, joint bones begin to die, a process known as aseptic necrosis. All these processes can and do produce pain, and the more of them that are operative, the worse the pain generally is.

From a broad perspective, pain and damage in OA result from an imbalance in degenerative and repair processes within the body, in which, finally, even the repair processes go wrong and contribute to the damage. Although cartilage is not innervated by nerve fibers capable of "feeling" pain, almost all other parts of synovial joints are richly innervated and thus quite capable of registering pain in response to the mechanical damage and low-grade inflammation that characterize OA joints. Moreover, even though cartilage lacks pain fibers, when it becomes inflamed, this inflammation spills over and activates pain-sensitive nerve endings in other parts of the joint, which generates a sensation of pain. The severity of pain correlates with radiologic findings of synovial inflammation and with bone changes within the joints. But as in all chronic pain conditions, the story doesn't stop at the site of injury. Rather, joint inflammation can lead to peripheral and central sensitization, a process we have described in response to many previous questions. In the case of OA, evidence suggests that when nerves become sensitized they may cause the release of inflammatory chemicals into the already damaged joint, which only worsens and perpetuates the pain and joint damage.

Although OA can affect any joint in the body that has a synovial membrane surrounding it, the disease most often impacts the knees, hips, hands, and spine. The primary causes of disability in OA are joint pain, joint stiffness, and limited joint mobility.

PART TWO

Neurobiology of Pain

Can you describe the pathways that conduct painful signals from the periphery of the body to the brain?

Can the brain change the intensity of pain?

Can chronic pain cause changes in the brain structure?

More . . .

41. Do genes play a role in chronic pain?

Chronic pain disorders are very diverse, making genetic research into their causes a daunting task. Many genes contribute to our ability to feel pain, and so not surprisingly, many genes have been found to be involved—at least to some degree—in a wide range of chronic pain disorders. Basically, most genes that produce chemicals or structures involved in how pain is experienced and processed in the brain or body seem to come in forms that are likely to protect against, or promote, the development of chronic pain. These different forms of the same gene are called "alleles." As one example of this, certain forms of the gene that code for opioid receptors (the sites of action for opiate medications) seem to increase the risk of developing a chronic pain disorder. Other genes that appear to be involved include those that contribute to nerve conduction and those that code for the production and signaling ability of neurotransmitters such as serotonin, norepinephrine, and dopamine. Because these neurotransmitters are often abnormal in major depression, it shouldn't come as a surprise that chronic pain conditions such as fibromyalgia appear to share many genetic risk factors with major depression. But associations don't stop there. Many of these genes are risk factors for many conditions that afflict people in the modern world, including anxiety disorders, bipolar disorder, attention deficit disorder, and cardiovascular disease. The fact that the same gene alleles increase the risk for so many conditions may help to explain why so many medical, psychiatric, and pain-related conditions tend to be comorbid with each other.

Allow us to give two more examples of how genes for pain disorders can overlap with other conditions.

Catechol-O-methyltransferase (COMT) is an enzyme that is important for breaking down serotonin, norepinephrine, and dopamine. Like all genes, it varies in its exact makeup from person to person. These differences are called polymorphisms. One polymorphism in the COMT gene has been shown to increase how sensitive people are to a painful stimulus and to have a reduced mu-opioid receptor response to pain. Remember that the opioid system is very important in dampening pain sensations, so this reduced receptor response may explain the increased pain sensation. It also shows how one system can affect another, given that COMT has no direct effect on opioid function. But don't think that this COMT polymorphism is unique to pain perception just because it affects it. Rather, this polymorphism has also been reported to increase the risk for a wide range of stress-related psychiatric conditions, including major depression, schizophrenia, anxiety disorders, and attention deficit hyperactivity disorder (ADHD).

A second gene that has polymorphisms that increase the risk of chronic pain (fibromyalgia in this case) is the one that codes for an important receptor for the neurotransmitter dopamine. Polymorphisms in this receptor (called the DRD4 receptor) also appear to increase the risk for ADHD. This is especially interesting given a recent large study showing that behavioral disturbances in childhood that are commonly associated with ADHD significantly increase the risk for chronic widespread pain in adulthood. In conclusion, given their substantial genetic overlap, it is not surprising that chronic pain and psychiatric disorders are so often comorbid or that they share so many emotional, cognitive, and physical symptoms.

Neurobiology of Pain

42. Can you describe pathways that conduct painful signals from the periphery of the body to the brain?

Let's walk through the entire process of how pain signals get to the brain. Let's use as an example hitting your thumb with a hammer while trying to hang a picture on the wall. The slamming of the hammer on the thumb produces significant mechanical pressure on the tissue of the thumb. This pressure activates pain sensors in the skin that translate this mechanical pressure into electrical impulses that are sent down small peripheral nerve fibers that have their cell bodies in an area adjacent to the spinal cord called the "dorsal root ganglia." (DRG). These DRG cells then send the signal on to secondary sensory neurons that reside within an area of the spinal cord known as the dorsal horn (see Figure 1). From the dorsal horn and the dorsal column, the neural message reflecting the hammer hitting the thumb is sent up the spinal cord to the brain by two semi-independent pathways, one of which is called the spinothalamic tract, and the other, which is called the spinoparabrachial tract. These two tracts end in various clusters of neurons in the brain called nuclei (see Figure 2). Most of the nuclei that first receive pain information from the periphery of the body (hammer hitting thumb in this case) are located in the thalamus, which lies deep in the brain and functions as the brain's primary relay station. The thalamus begins processing the pain signals coming up from the spinal cord and then forwards the message on to a large number of brain areas that will help to locate where the pain is, to assess how painful and dangerous it is, and then help to move the body out of harm's way. Sometimes a picture is worth a thousand words, and this is certainly the case for trying to visualize complex pathways we've just described. To help you better understand how pain gets from the periphery of the body up to the brain; take a close look at Figures 2 and 5.

43. What is the role of the brain in perceiving and responding to pain?

This question takes up where the last one left off, which is in the thalamus, the primary relay station for the brain. So, let's continue and provide more detail about how the brain registers and responds to a painful stimulus from the periphery of the body, such as the hammer that hit the thumb in Question 42. The easiest way to think about how the brain registers pain is to ask yourself why pain is important and what the brain needs to do to make best use of the information. The simplest reason pain is important is because it is a signal that you are in a dangerous situation that could result in damage to your body. Pain should be able to powerfully grab our attention, because whether we live or die may depend on how we respond. Thus, it is not surprising that pain powerfully activates an area of the brain called the limbic system, which "fires off" in response to danger of all kinds. When the limbic areas of the brain become rapidly active, people generally feel startled, anxious, frightened, and the like. These feelings are unpleasant but important, because they force us to stop what we are doing and pay close attention to the danger. But to do this well, we need to know where the danger is, so it makes sense that the thalamus directs the pain signal up to an area of the brain known as the somatosensory cortex. This is the part of the brain that is able to specifically locate which part of the body nerve impulses are coming from. Together, these brain areas are frequently viewed as forming a "pain matrix" in the brain. This is a useful concept because as we'll see, activity in this matrix tends to be abnormal in many patients with chronic pain conditions (see Figure 5).

Neurobiology of Pain

In addition to the brain regions that have been discussed thus far, the thalamus also directs pain signals coming from the body up to the frontal lobes of the brain, which are also included in the brain's "pain matrix." These brain regions do several things of direct relevance to dealing with the danger that pain often indicates. First, the frontal lobes control bodily movement, so it is important that the pain message gets to these brain areas so the affected part of the body can be moved out of harm's way. Second, the frontal lobes are involved in long-range planning and placing individual events in larger contexts related to a person's long-term goals. Third, frontal regions, especially regions in the middle of the frontal lobes, play important roles in activating the body's stress response systems (i.e., the HPA axis and autonomic nervous system). Given that pain often means we are in a "fight-or-flight" situation, this stress system activation makes a good deal of sense (see Figures 5 and 6).

Let's summarize what we know about how the frontal lobes deal with pain by revisiting our example of the hammer striking the thumb while hanging a picture. If this happens while we are alone, the frontal lobes see no problem with allowing us to curse and rapidly drop the picture. But suppose we are hanging the picture in the apartment of a man or woman we very much want to start dating and thus want to make a good impression. Now the frontal lobes interpret the situation quite differently and decide that our long-term goals are better achieved by suppressing the urge to drop the picture and curse, acting instead as if nothing much has happened that would show our ineptitude with a hammer and nail! Nonetheless, despite our cool exterior, not even our desire to make a good social impression will be enough to keep our frontal lobes from activating the body's stress systems, with the result that our heart rate and blood pressure will go up.

Many chronic pain conditions have been found to be associated with altered functioning in the brain's pain matrix. Let's take fibromyalgia (FM) as an example. Studies have found that brain areas in the pain matrix respond to non-painful stimuli the way these brain areas respond to painful stimuli in normal people. One study found that individuals without FM required twice the pain stimulus as FM patients to get an equivalent amount of activation in the brain's pain matrix (see Figure 5).

In summary, our best evidence suggests that brain regions involved in processing sensory, emotional, and cognitive aspects of pain (also known as the pain matrix) play key roles in how we perceive and respond to pain. Many studies have now shown that these areas function abnormally in many patients with chronic pain conditions, and these functional abnormalities play an important role in the disorders themselves. More than this, because the pain matrix often functions abnormally when people are under psychological stress, this may help explain why pain disorders and psychiatric conditions so frequently co-occur.

44. Can the brain change the intensity of pain?

It is true! The brain has the ability to both increase and decrease the intensity of pain signals coming from the body. Whether the brain does one or the other can profoundly impact how an individual perceives any given painful event. Neuroimaging studies have consistently found that chronic pain conditions such as fibromyalgia and neuropathic pain (NeP) are characterized by abnormalities in the function of pain-processing areas in the brain that play primary roles in either inhibiting or amplifying the perception of pain. Brain areas important for

Many chronic pain conditions have been found to be associated with altered functioning in the brain's pain matrix.

Neurobiology of Pain

inhibiting activity in pain pathways coming from the body include the anterior cingulate, insula, and several brain stem nuclei (see Figures 2 and 5). The anterior cingulate also appears to play an important role in modulating pathways so that the brain is able to amplify pain signals coming from the body.

Norepinephrine, serotonin, and acetylcholine are the principal neurotransmitters in *inhibitory* pathways that descend from the brain to the body. Primary neurotransmitters in descending pathways from the brain to the body that amplify pain perception (called *facilitatory* pathways) include serotonin, neurotensin, cholecystokinins, and brain-derived neurotrophic factor (BDNF). Abnormal functioning in descending pain pathways, either as a result of inadequate activity in the inhibitory pathway or increased activity in the facilitatory pathway, or a combination of both, appears to play an important role in the development of a number of strange pain symptoms seen in many chronic pain conditions associated with central sensitization (see Figure 2). These symptoms include allodynia, the perception of pain in response to light touch, and hyperalgesia, a generalized tendency to experience pain as especially unpleasant or intense.

45. Can chronic pain cause changes in the brain structure?

In addition to functional differences, several studies have found significant structural changes in the brains of chronic pain patients. For example, a recent study reported that patients with fibromyalgia have significant reductions in the volume of a number of brain areas when compared to individuals of the same age and sex without FM. Brain areas that appear to be "shrunken" in FM include the cingulate cortex, insula, medial prefrontal cortex (mPFC), and parahippocampal lobe of the brain. This study also found that the longer people had FM, the smaller these brain areas were, with the result that each year of the illness had an impact equivalent to 9.5 times the loss of brain matter that occurs as a result of normal aging. Similar results have been found in patients with chronic back pain and no significant symptoms of depression. One study in this population found significantly reduced volume in two areas of the brain, the dorsolateral prefrontal cortex and the thalamus. Moreover, volume loss in the dorsolateral prefrontal cortex was associated with increased intensity and duration of pain symptoms. As in FM, the magnitude of volume reduction in the gray matter of the brain in chronic back pain patients was equivalent to 10 to 20 years of normal aging. Finally, many studies now show that changes in the structure and function of the brain may also account for many of the abnormalities in thinking and feeling that often accompany chronic pain conditions such as FM.

On learning this type of information, our patient Susan said:

This information was eye-opening and provides motivation for me to do whatever it takes to effectively and consistently manage my pain issues.

46. Are trigger points and tender points one and the same?

Trigger points are defined as nodules in muscles that can be felt and that have clearly defined margins. Researchers believe that they are caused by contractions in muscle tissue. Trigger points are tender and irritable. Applying pressure to them causes the muscle to twitch and produces pain at their site and often other nearby

Neurobiology of Pain

Trigger points
Specific points in our body that, when irritated, cause pain in other parts of the body. Doctors will often look for these points to inject pain medication in order to reduce pain.

areas of the body. Although trigger points are clearly definable and observable, little is known about their origin. Pressure on a trigger point typically reproduces pain similar to the pain a patient typically complains about. Generally, the pattern of pain that radiates from the trigger point coincides with the surface of the involved muscle. Most of the time, no clear medical cause (such as infection, cancer, or tissue trauma) is found to account for why any given trigger point exists or why it causes such pain. However, whatever the origin, trigger points are most frequently found in the context of myofascial pain disorder.

Tender points are discreet areas in the body at which applied pressure produces significant pain, but tender points are not characterized by the presence of a definable nodule or other physical abnormality. Tender points are a central diagnostic feature of fibromyalgia. To make a diagnosis of FM, the American College of Rheumatology (ACR) criteria require the presence of pain in response to pressure applied to at least 11 out of 18 anatomically defined tender points. Most FM patients will have numerous tender points coinciding with muscle–tendon junctions. However, these tender points are not fixed. In fact, patients will have an increase in tender points when under stress or deprived of sleep. Thus, the number and location of tender points tends to fluctuate with time. Although most tender points are located in muscle tissue, some are not, although they are found in close proximity to tendon insertion points. Finally, despite the distinctions we've described, some researchers believe that trigger points and tender points have more commonalities than differences and that distinctions between the two may be overrated in the clinical literature.

47. I've heard a lot about chronic pain affecting the hypothalamic–pituitary–adrenal (HPA) axis. Can you tell me about this?

Although the literature is somewhat unclear, it appears that chronic pain disorders have a significant impact on the function of **hypothalamic–pituitary–adrenal (HPA) axis**. Most studies report that conditions of chronic pain, fatigue, and other somatic symptoms (e.g., FM, Chronic Fatigue Syndrome [CFS]) are characterized by decreased production of the primary HPA axis hormone, which is cortisol. However, these studies also often report that the receptors for cortisol in the body have increased sensitivity in chronic pain conditions. This has left researchers to puzzle over whether the increased sensitivity of the receptors compensates for the decreased production of cortisol or overcompensates for the low cortisol production.

However, not all studies find that cortisol receptors are overly sensitive in chronic pain disorders. In fact, a number of studies have found that the cortisol receptors are not sensitive enough! Why these contradictions should exist in the scientific literature is not clear, but we have a bias in favor of the possibility that cortisol receptors may be underfunctioning in the context of chronic pain. We have this bias for several reasons. First, major depression—which is very frequently comorbid with chronic pain—is often associated with reduced cortisol sensitivity. Second, a large recent study found that how resistant people were to cortisol, strongly predicted their likelihood of having a new onset of chronic widespread pain in the succeeding 15 months. Third, a recent treatment study of patients with FM found that symptomatic improvements as a result of therapeutic intervention were associated with increases—rather than decreases—in cortisol signaling. Fourth, cortisol is

Hypothalamic–pituitary–adrenal (HPA) axis

Neuroendocrine system composed of several interrelated components (hypothalamus, pituitary, and adrenal glands).

Neurobiology of Pain

profoundly anti-inflammatory, yet chronic pain conditions are usually characterized by increased inflammation, suggesting that cortisol signaling is insufficient. Finally, if chronic pain conditions such as FM and CFS were caused in part by too much cortisol activity, one would expect that treating these patients with cortisol or similar hormones would worsen their condition. In fact, several studies show that treatment with cortisol or similar hormones actually improves a number of symptoms that are common in chronic pain conditions.

Less controversial than whether cortisol signaling is excessive or impaired in the context of pain, is the consistent finding that pain disorders are characterized by abnormalities in the daily rhythm of cortisol production. Specifically, patients with FM and CFS (as well as depression and a number of medical conditions associated with pain and fatigue) tend to show a flattening of the daily cortisol rhythm in contrast to healthy individuals who typically demonstrate high cortisol in the morning that falls throughout the day and into the evening. Flattening of the cortisol rhythm is an ominous finding indeed, given that it predicts subsequent development of chronic widespread pain in medically healthy individuals. As you might predict, behavioral interventions that improve pain symptoms in FM patients also steepen the cortisol slope.

48. Can chronic pain be associated with changes in autonomic nervous system function?

Yes. In fact, alterations in the autonomic nervous system, or ANS, are among the most repeated abnormalities seen in chronic pain conditions. Although we've discussed the ANS in previous questions, let's do a quick review. The ANS is called autonomic as in "automatic," meaning that it innervates many bodily functions that are usually seen as beyond conscious control, such as heart rate and digestion. The ANS is also very much involved in both stress responses and rest and recuperation. The stress arm of the ANS is called the sympathetic nervous system. When it is activated, heart rate goes up, blood pressure increases, and attention narrows to whatever appears to be the source of danger. This is the famous "fight-or-flight" response that provides energy and focus to help an organism react optimally to dangerous situations. The other arm of the ANS is called the parasympathetic nervous system. This system is in many ways the opposite of the sympathetic system. The parasympathetic system lowers heart rate and blood pressure, enhances digestion, and induces feelings of relaxation and trust that promote social interaction.

Given these descriptions you can probably guess that many chronic pain conditions appear to be characterized by imbalances between the two arms of the ANS. In addition to contributing to symptoms themselves, these types of imbalances also contribute to HPA axis and inflammatory abnormalities seen in chronic pain. For example, in a study of men with FM, abnormal blood pressure and heart rate changes upon standing up for long periods indicated sympathetic hyperactivity and a concomitant reduction in parasympathetic tone. Several other authors have identified sympathetic hyperactivity as a component of the stress response that both causes and maintains FM and NeP symptoms such as fatigue, sleep disturbance, anxiety, depression, and gastrointestinal problems. Studies suggest that inflammation is increased in chronic pain conditions, and patients with chronic pain respond to inflammation with increased sympathetic activity. To close the loop, chronic pain patients have also been shown to experience more pain than normal people when injected with norepinephrine, which is the primary neurotransmitter of the sympathetic nervous system. This suggests that for any given amount of inflammation, patients with chronic pain will produce more norepinephrine, and for every unit of norepinephrine produced will experience more pain!

In addition to its association with pain symptoms, the ANS may also offer promise as an avenue for treatment. For example, recent research shows that biofeedback training designed to decrease sympathetic activity and increase parasympathetic tone in patients with FM is effective in reducing pain symptoms.

49. What is the relationship between chronic pain and immunity?

Pain, much like stress, is associated with activation of systems in the brain and body that work together to help us best deal with the types of acute danger that were most likely to cause either stress or pain during human evolution. As much as we don't like pain, and as damaging as the physical changes that accompany chronic pain can be, it is important to recognize that pain exists because it provided a strong survival advantage across millions of years of evolution. Like psychological stress, pain activates the HPA axis and sympathetic nervous system, as well as the body's inflammatory pathways. Each of these systems plays an important role in helping an organism cope with danger and return to normal functioning. But like many other good things, these systems can go bad, and they do so in patients with chronic pain.

In the last several questions we have discussed the role of the HPA axis and autonomic nervous system in the development and maintenance of chronic pain. Now it is time to discuss the immune system, which is every bit as much a part of the "fight-or-flight" response as the HPA axis or the ANS. It is no surprise then, that virtually every kind of chronic pain is associated with altered immune function and/or increased inflammation. In fact, in some painful conditions such as postherpetic neuralgia, multiple sclerosis, radiculopathies, neuropathic pain, and FM, inflammation may well be the key abnormality driving the disorder. In other pain conditions, such as osteoarthritis, inflammatory components are less obvious but nevertheless essential in pain development.

We have talked a lot in this book about central sensitization, a process by which nerve cells become more and more sensitive to pain stimuli. Immune responses to damaged tissue, with concomitant release of inflammatory chemicals, play a central role in peripheral sensitization, which in turn promotes central sensitization. But inflammation doesn't just cause central sensitization. These processes can reverse themselves such, that nerves coming out of the spinal cord can drive inflammation in peripheral tissues, leading to even more pain signals coming from the damaged tissue. Cells in the central nervous system called microglia are able to produce inflammatory chemicals in response to signals of tissue damage in the body. Researchers are increasingly recognizing that these central nervous system inflammatory cells play a key role in fostering central sensitization and in the changes in brain structure that ensue in the context of chronic pain.

Increased inflammation in the blood and in the fluid surrounding the brain has been repeatedly cited as a shared feature of chronic pain conditions such as FM,

NeP, and CFS that are characterized by pain, fatigue, sleep disturbances, and cognitive complaints. Many studies have reported elevations in a number of inflammatory signaling chemicals called cytokines. One of these, interleukin-8 (IL-8) has been repeatedly observed to be elevated in people with FM. IL-8 is released by the pain promoting peptide substance P, and it is known to modulate HPA axis activity and induce sympathetically mediated pain. Moreover, several studies find associations between blood levels of IL-8 and subjective pain ratings in FM. In addition to elevations in inflammatory activity, studies increasingly suggest that chronic pain conditions may also be caused by reductions in anti-inflammatory activity. For example, chronic widespread pain has been shown to be associated with reduced gene expression and blood protein levels of the anti-inflammatory cytokines IL-4 and IL-10.

In summary, altered neuroimmune signaling at every level of the nervous system has a major role in generating and perpetuating pain. The relationship between pain and inflammation unfortunately tends to be bidirectional, such that increased pain drives inflammation and inflammation increases pain.

50. What is the role of gender in chronic pain?

There are clear gender differences in the frequency of several chronic pain conditions, including fibromyalgia, neuropathic pain, multiple sclerosis–related pain, temporomandibular joint (TMJ) pain, and migraine headaches, just to name a few. Common features of these conditions include sensitivity to stress and evidence of increased inflammation. Links between susceptibility to stress and gender have been extensively studied in relation to depressive and anxiety disorders, both of which are highly comorbid with chronic pain conditions. Women are three times more likely to develop both depression and FM, and stress is a shared risk and etiological factor for both conditions. It is possible that because of augmented stress responses, women have a greater risk for all the stress-related disorders such as chronic pain and depression.

Women are three times more likely to develop both depression and FM.

Recent studies suggest another connection between gender and pain. Women appear to more readily activate inflammatory pathways in response to environmental adversity or injury. Inflammation, in turn, is modulated by estrogen. A recent study has found that women suffering from FM have significantly lower estrogen levels, despite elevated follicular-stimulating hormone (FSH), which promotes estrogen production. Therefore, insufficient regulation of inflammation by estrogen combined with more readily activated stress responses may contribute to greater prevalence of some chronic pain disorders in women.

Recent neuroimaging studies have demonstrated greater activation in multiple components of the central nervous system pain matrix (e.g., contralateral thalamus, insula, and parts of the prefrontal cortex) in response to experimentally induced pain in women when compared to men (see Figure 5). A tendency to focus on and exaggerate the threat value of painful stimuli and to negatively evaluate one's ability to cope (often referred to as "catastrophizing") is more common in women and appears to partially mediate the gender-pain relationship. Finally, studies suggest that while women are more likely to experience an increase in pain over the course of the day, men are more likely than women to have negative mood in the morning after an evening of increased pain.

Neurobiology of Pain

PART THREE

Non-Pharmacological Strategies for Pain Treatment

How do non-medication approaches work to control my chronic pain, and which ones are the most effective?

How can cognitive-behavioral therapy work for chronic pain?

What about physical exercise? Can it help?

More . . .

51. How do non-medication approaches work to control my chronic pain, and which ones are the most effective?

Non-medication approaches to controlling pain are a very important issue. As you have already discovered from reading the previous questions and answers in this book, chronic pain is a bio-psycho-social phenomenon, in which the body, brain, and mind all play important roles in controlling the amount of pain we feel. Many of the non-medication approaches we will talk about have demonstrated positive effects on one or more of the following: body, brain, and mind. Let's discuss this in more detail.

Scientific advances in the last two decades have shown that the mind affects the body and the body affects the mind. In fact, this link is so strong that a whole new school of thought looks at chronic pain as a mind–body disorder. As you already know, chronic pain is created and maintained by, among other things, pro-pain neurotransmitters, rewired pain circuitry, and our mental state (which typically indicates our level of stress, anxiety, and/or depression). While medications clearly play a role in reversing some of these issues, thereby reducing chronic pain, non-medication approaches have shown similar positive effects on pain. This is exciting news for both the medical community as well as the community of chronic pain sufferers! So to answer how these treatments work is best and most accurately answered by appreciating that non-medication treatments can powerfully alter brain and body chemicals that can cause pain relief. There is nothing hypothetical in what we are saying. Clinical published evidence clearly supports this thinking.

Now let's talk specifics. Physical exercise, which we will discuss in more detail later has shown positive effects on brain chemicals related to pain as well as pain outcomes. This physical exercise can be self-directed, or as directed by a physical therapist. Meditation similarly has demonstrated positive effects on both pain and anxiety and stress levels. **Cognitive-behavioral therapy (CBT)** is another very significant non-pharmacological intervention for chronic pain. This type of psychotherapy was originally developed for the treatment of depression. However, recent data show that chronic pain patients also benefit from harnessing the power of thoughts and behaviors in tapping down on chronic pain. For this reason, CBT is increasingly a part of chronic pain clinics, and referral to trained CBT therapists can usually be obtained by calling a pain clinic in your area or by being a patient at such a clinic.

It is our collective belief that *all* patients with chronic pain should be receiving non-pharmacological therapies, either by themselves or in combination with medication therapy. In the latter situation, there is most likely added benefit to receiving both forms of treatments. While most pain clinicians are well aware of non-pharmacological treatments and will readily recommend them for you, not all do so. It then becomes your responsibility, should your clinician not offer you such options, to actively engage your physician in a discussion on the topic of whether non-pharmacological treatments might be of assistance to you and what type would best meet your needs. One final comment: non-pharmacological treatments work best if they are applied on a regular basis for long periods of time. So, please avail yourself of the benefits of appropriate non-pharmacological treatments as you journey toward improvement in your chronic pain!

Cognitive-behavioral therapy (CBT)
Originally developed to help treat patients with depression, this therapy teaches patients to harness the power of their thoughts and change their behaviors to improve their mood and functioning.

Non-pharmacological treatments work best if they are applied on a regular basis for long periods of time.

52. What is "learned helplessness," and what role can it play in the psychological lives of people with chronic pain?

Helplessness is a feeling of despair in which one's outlook is negative, dark, and pessimistic, suffused with the belief that he or she can't be helped. Sometimes, as a result of physical adversities such as chronic pain or emotional adversities such as sexual abuse, physical or mental abuse, depression, anxiety, and/or stress, a person comes to believe that things will never get better. That develops into a feeling of helplessness that can solidify into a constant belief system. This is then termed as "**learned helplessness**."

Learned helplessness

As a result of physical (chronic pain), or emotional adversities (sexual abuse, physical or mental abuse, depression, anxiety, and/or stress), a person comes to believe that things will never get better. Consequently, feelings of helplessness may progress and solidify into a constant belief system.

This is a dangerous belief system, as it does not serve you well. Now, please don't get us wrong—we are not suggesting that learned helplessness is of your choosing or that you might even be fully aware of it. In fact, learned helplessness is a sneaky cognitive belief system that insidiously burrows into your thoughts in such a way that you don't even know it is there. It is, however, hugely damaging to both mental health and recovery from chronic pain. It is well worth your while to explore your thoughts, either by yourself or with the help of a trained therapist or clinician, to ensure you don't have elements of learned helplessness. If you do, it is worth your while to change these ideas.

You may think that this is more easily said than done, and that if we had the kind of pain you have, we too would be feeling helpless! We agree this is a potentially difficult issue, especially if you have a significant chronic pain problem. But the payoffs are large, so we urge you to explore your thoughts to find any evidence of learned helplessness. Consider posing these questions to yourself:

Do I believe that the chronic pain rules my life? Do I have control over it or does it control me? Do I have hope that I will get better? Do I believe even if my chronic pain doesn't go away, I can still flourish in life?

If you find, after asking yourself these questions, that you may have elements of learned helplessness as a result of chronic pain and/or mental stress, definitely seek counseling. CBT therapy (which is discussed elsewhere in this book) is a particularly good way to challenge these negative, unproductive, harmful thought patterns. Also, joining a pain support group might be of help to you.

53. How can cognitive-behavioral therapy work for chronic pain?

At multiple places in this book, you will note that we talk about cognitive-behavioral therapy. Let's have a more complete discussion on this issue now. First, what is CBT? Cognitive-behavioral therapy is a form of psychotherapy that was created by psychiatrist Dr. Aaron Beck a few decades ago to help patients suffering from depression. The premise was that depression is often caused by faulty and inaccurate thinking patterns and behaviors. Dr. Beck believed that once we recognize these thought and behavior patterns as problematic, we change them, which causes the depression to diminish. This is not a form of unconditional positive thinking, but rather correct, realistic thinking. Cognitive-behavioral therapy has now been demonstrated quite conclusively to work for depression and anxiety disorders.

Recent research shows the same is true for many pain disorders too. Pain, particularly chronic pain, can often change our view of self, the future, and the world.

Pain, particularly chronic pain, can often change our view of self, the future, and the world.

Non-Pharmacological Strategies for Pain Treatment

This can lead to feelings of despair, stress, helplessness, anxiety, and depression. Often led by a trained therapist, CBT offers people suffering with chronic pain an opportunity to examine their thoughts and beliefs and assess if they are realistic or faulty. If they are the latter, the CBT therapist then offers suggestions and ideas on how these thoughts might be changed. Research has shown that this process not only helps with mood and life outlook, but also with pain. Even more encouragingly, CBT has now been demonstrated to help even after formal therapy is completed. In other words, skills learned in CBT training frequently stay with the person and lead to long-term improvement.

Be aware that many pain clinicians are not fully aware of CBT's benefits, and you may need to initiate a conversation with them on this topic. Be persistent in asking for their thoughts on CBT and to whom might they refer you. Once you are referred, you may want to confirm with the CBT therapist by calling the office to make sure that he or she is comfortable working with chronic pain patients—a surprisingly large number of therapists don't have the training to work with chronic pain patients or choose not to work with them. Checking his or her credentials is also a good idea. Your prospective therapist should have at least a master's degree in psychology, counseling, or social work, and have formal training in CBT. Don't be shy about asking all the questions you may have, as a good fit between you and your CBT therapist is crucial.

In closing, we might add that CBT appears to be a significant investment for you in terms of both time and money. But in most cases, it is well worth your while. Please do discuss this issue with your clinician.

54. My doctor told me that I "catastrophize" too much and that it is making my pain worse. What does she mean and what can I do about it?

We wish your doctor had phrased it differently or fully explained to you what was meant by that statement, but let us first discuss what the medical profession means by "catastrophizing." It is a term used to describe the human tendency to sometimes see things as if "the sky is falling." As you can imagine, when someone has chronic pain, it is easy for that person to fall into the trap of unconditionally believing that their pain will never be better, that they will never be functional at all, that they will lose their job, or that everyone will abandon them. In most situations, these beliefs are neither accurate nor logical. Yet a person having these belief patterns on a regular basis truly believes them and is said to catastrophize excessively or unproductively.

So why would your doctor be concerned about this trait? There is a simple reason—catastrophizing reduces the quality of life, increases the chance of developing depression and/or anxiety, and most importantly, worsens pain control. So, for all these reasons, it is valuable for you to assess yourself through your own eyes, through your family and friends' eyes, and through your doctor's opinion to see if you catastrophize. If you do, it behooves you to take the corrective steps.

These corrective steps start with the realization that this tendency is part of how you cope with pain, and that catastrophizing worsens your control over pain. This is not what you want. As it is often difficult to self-correct this tendency, we recommend you seek help. This could be the help of your clinician, your pastoral counselor, a good friend, or even a trained counselor. The catastrophizing trait is a long-standing one, so it is possible that you may not even be aware that you do it. In your mind, this might be the only way to look at your situation. That's why asking others to assess you is valuable. In the long run, you will benefit significantly from attacking this trait, should you possess it.

55. What about physical exercise? Can it help?

Yes, physical exercise can be helpful in many kinds of chronic pain, but an immediate word of caution is needed at this point. Please seek your physician's advice if you are about to embark on any new exercise program.

Over the last 5 years, advances in molecular biology have shown us that exercise appears to improve our health at the cellular and even the subcellular levels (inside the cell). This is remarkable information. Physical exercise appears to strengthen our innate pain modulating mechanisms. There are now studies that clearly demonstrate the pain-controlling effects of physical exercise in patients with fibromyalgia, low back pain, osteoarthritis of knee joint pain, and so forth. This evidence is quite strong and has been reliably replicated.

So, the decision is in: exercise can be helpful in chronic pain, either by itself or combined with other treatment modalities. If you have had chronic pain for a while, it is quite possible you have actually been avoiding physical exercise. This is perhaps because exercise made the pain worse, or you were tired and fatigued a lot and you learned to avoid exercise. It's important to reverse this trend. No doubt exercise is good for your mind and body, so now it is time to accept that exercise is good for chronic pain too. As to which exercise to choose and how to increase the amount, you really should work with your clinician to determine this. Pain should by itself not be an excuse to not exercise. There is almost always a type of exercise that you can engage in (walking, biking, water-based exercise, etc.), so there are no excuses. We recommend you make exercise a regular part of your life, today, tomorrow, and for years to come!

56. I have been hearing about meditation being helpful in pain management. Could you tell me more?

You have indeed heard this correctly. **Meditation** has now been shown in some studies to actually change the levels of our pain-processing chemicals. At this point, you may be asking yourself—what is meditation? Well, while there are multiple types of meditation techniques, all of them are techniques to calm and focus the mind. It appears that meditation helps both the mind and the body. This is exciting and new information, but we have to temper this excitement with the recognition that really rigorous research into meditation is just now starting. Because of this, there are still a lot of unanswered questions, such as what kind of meditation is best for pain control, how long you should practice every day, and so forth.

Meditation

A contemplative process whereby an individual attempts to get beyond reflexive thinking into a state of more profound awareness and relaxation.

Having said this, we still believe that as someone afflicted with chronic pain, you should look into meditation. Striking evidence reveals that meditation is a true mind–body experience, and meditation appears to reduce our body's inflammatory response that increases our pain. Meditation is also known to positively impact the autonomic nervous system and other stress-modulating systems, so meditation may be useful at multiple levels.

It can also help to distract you from pain and to learn coping skills.

As most cities now have meditation/yoga classes, we encourage you to take some of these classes to begin experimenting with meditation. You can also seek resources over the Internet. It is important for you to remember that to achieve maximum benefit from meditation, you should practice it regularly. Long-term practitioners appear to derive the most benefits.

Sue said:

I've found meditation to be a great intervention not only for physical well-being but also emotional health. I attended a 3-day Qigong workshop last summer—one aspect of Qigong is meditation. The results were impressive. The key to getting the most out of Qigong or any meditation is consistency. This is a struggle for me, but the benefits of regular Qigong practice make it worth the effort.

57. Can acupuncture help me?

While none of us are acupuncture practitioners, we have referred patients for this form of treatment. Like anything else for the management of chronic pain, this technique is highly effective for some and not for others. Don't let this discourage you from at least exploring this form of chronic pain treatment as an option for your chronic pain condition.

Acupuncture

An ancient Chinese pain treatment in which needles are inserted and then manipulated along meridians where, according to Chinese texts, body energy flows.

Acupuncture is an ancient Chinese pain treatment in which needles are inserted and then manipulated along meridians where, according to Chinese texts, body energy flows. There is a fairly large amount of scientific literature supporting acupuncture's effectiveness. In fact, we encourage you to visit a website maintained by a branch of the National Institute of Medicine—the National Center for Complementary and Alternative Medicine (http://nccam.nih.gov/health/acupuncture/). This is a highly trusted scientific body, and you will benefit from visiting its informational site on acupuncture. In addition to reading materials, there are educational videos on this site that are worthy of your time and energy.

Another recommended source is the American Academy of Medical Acupuncture website (www.medicalacupuncture.org), which has a great deal of useful information as well as the means for you to get a referral in your local area. Some health insurance programs are beginning to pay for acupuncture services, and we recommend that you call your own insurance carrier to check to see if yours does, too.

Acupuncture appears to be effective above and beyond a placebo effect. Some studies have indicated that acupuncture can alter endogenous opioid levels that can help us with pain. Science has not yet unlocked the mysteries of how acupuncture works or which type of patient it is most likely to benefit. While we wait for these scientific advances to occur, we encourage you to explore acupuncture as a possible treatment for your chronic pain condition.

Acupuncture appears to be effective above and beyond a placebo effect.

Sue said:

I used acupuncture before and after all my surgeries. The results were amazing. I consistently experienced reduction in pain and increased range of motion. I believe having an expectation that acupuncture will be helpful is crucial to success. I think going into it with the right attitude and expectations made the intervention more effective.

58. Is there a diet that can help with my chronic pain?

While there is no solid scientific evidence that any particular diet can help with your chronic pain, we are glad you are considering the impact of nutrition in your life as you deal with this pain.

As indicated in previous sections of this book, chronic pain by itself is a state of toxicity in your body, with significant changes occurring in your body's autonomic nervous, endocrine system, and inflammatory systems. All of these add to stress and wear and tear on your body, which can adversely affect your physical health and may lead to weight gain, glucose changes, and lipid changes. Thus, counteracting these changes by thinking about your diet is a very good idea.

There are additional reasons for examining your nutritional habits and making appropriate changes is a good idea. Obesity is now an American epidemic. We know that greater weight on a person increases the risk of developing arthritis. Thus, losing weight through sensible changes in diet and exercise could directly help with chronic pain. Evidence also suggests that medications are generally less effective in people who have a weight issue, providing even more reasons for you to carefully examine your diet.

Consider asking yourself these questions:

- Do I eat a nutritionally sound diet?
- Do I ingest the right amount of calories to maintain my weight at a healthy level?
- Do I overeat certain kinds of food?
- Do I need to ask for help in readjusting my diet (such as consulting a nutritionist, joining an organization such as Weight Watchers, etc.)?

- Do I know, with the help of my primary care doctor, what my fasting blood sugars and lipids are?
- Do I have a plan to counteract any problems I have detected?

Please remember, should you detect a negative area, you are not alone in your attempts to solve these problems. Your healthcare team is more than capable of helping you, so reach out to them for help!

We have some excellent resources to point you toward. We recommend that you calculate your body mass index at the following website: http://www.nhlbisupport. com/bmi. **Body mass index (BMI)** is a measure that will allow you to see whether you are at optimum weight. We recommend you calculate yours now and then perhaps recalculate it every 6 months or so, to make sure that you are not drifting in the wrong weight direction. Another wonderful site to use to learn about good, balanced nutrition is the U.S. Department of Agriculture's website: www. mypyramid.gov. We have found it to be an excellent educational website that you can visit again and again as you watch your diet as a means of conquering chronic pain.

Body mass index (BMI)

A measure based on weight and body surface, often used as an indicator of obesity.

59. I hear that doctors specializing in physical medicine and rehabilitation can help me with my pain. What can they do for me?

You have heard correctly. In the last few years, physicians who specialize in **physical medicine and rehabilitation (PMR)** have stepped up to the plate to help chronic pain patients. PMR is a well-recognized medical specialty that requires physicians to spend several years in residency training after graduating from medical school. These physicians are exceptionally well-trained in helping patients with limited movements

Physical medicine and rehabilitation (PMR)

A medical specialty, practiced by physicians who are exceptionally well-trained in helping patients with limitations imposed by strokes, head injuries, cardiovascular disease, muscle, bone, joint and soft tissue injury. Physical medicine specialists have significant expertise in helping patients with chronic pain.

secondary to strokes, head injuries, and so forth, but they also have significant expertise in helping patients with chronic pain even without the above-mentioned conditions. They are well-trained in the art of diagnosing musculoskeletal pain and are used to working on multidisciplinary teams. They are also becoming more familiar and comfortable with prescribing physical therapy to assist in pain reduction and are gaining more expertise in interventional pain control (i.e., where a needle is used to block nerves, etc.).

Now, not every PMR physician works with patients with chronic pain, so it is advisable before you go to see such a clinician that you inquire regarding his or her expertise. In general, we have found PMR physicians to be well-trained, well-balanced pain clinicians who often use pharmacological and non-pharmacological treatments in wise combinations. Should you go see one after checking out their background and clinical expertise, you likely will have a good experience. It is always wise to see if your clinician is board certified and has no significant problems with your state's medical board. This is easily done by searching the Internet for the name of your state's medical regulatory board, and then searching for the physician's name there. It will give you a quick history of any disciplinary problems that might have been reported. Because of their background, these types of clinicians are also valuable members of your pain management team.

60. Every time I have tried to exercise, I hurt more. I have come to believe that I should avoid exercise to stop my pain from becoming worse. Am I making the right decision?

Your decision to try to exercise is certainly correct, though the way you might be doing it is perhaps incorrect. Allow us to explain.

First, let's examine the research data on pain and exercise. The overwhelming finding is that exercise helps reduce pain. Exercise appears to strengthen "the brakes" on our body's pain-processing pathways. However, many chronic pain patients have unconditioned bodies as a result of not having exercised for long periods of time. When they pick up exercise where they left off before they developed chronic pain, their pain worsens. This is a common and untreatable mistake made by chronic pain patients.

The over-whelming finding is that exercise helps reduce pain.

There are ways to overcome this barrier. First, it is important to accept the fact that exercise is a valuable thing to do for our body, mind, and pain management. Second, accept the fact that you should start a very gradual exercise program. Start slowly and build up slowly, but keep going—this ought to be the motto of your exercise plan.

You may want to start out with non-weight–bearing forms of exercise such as bicycling or water-based exercise. This is a particularly good option for those with fibromyalgia, arthritis of the knee or ankle, or hip pain. Build things up very gradually. Remember this: it is better to exercise at lower intensity for short durations, as long as you exercise regularly, than to overdo the exercise and suffer a disheartening increase in pain. The intensity can always be built up gradually, but if pain worsens as a result of overaggressive duration or intensity of exercise, then the chronic pain patient learns the wrong lesson—"Exercise hurts me more, therefore I shouldn't do it." This is an incorrect but understandable response.

It is our belief that nearly all individuals with chronic pain should exercise. Don't make the mistake of being too aggressive with your exercise program; start slowly, but keep building upward. Exercise is one of the great forms of helping your mind, body, and pain, but you must do it the right way—the way that best suits your particular situation!

Sue said:

I guess I'm like everyone else because after my surgeries I resumed my exercise routine with unreasonable expecta- tions—heavy weights, resulting in increased pain. Gradu- ally I cut my exercise back to almost nothing, resulting in even less mobility and range of motion. I've had to start from scratch, resetting my expectations and starting out slow as I increase my strength. I always feel better when I'm active.

61. What is a "placebo" pain response?

When researchers conduct research trials with medica- tions, they often conduct what are called double-blind trials. In a double-blind, placebo-controlled trial, some patients get the actual medication, while others get a dummy pill that does not contain any medication, also called a **placebo**. Typically, neither the researchers nor the patient know what is in the pill that any given patient is taking. Usually there is a 50% chance the pill has active medication and a 50% chance that the med- ication is a look-alike that contains an inactive sub- stance.

Placebo

A dummy pill (most often starch) that does not contain the medication; it is often used in con- trolled trials for new medications.

In such trials, quite often some patients who are on med- ications improve. This would, of course, be expected. However, often some patients on placebo also improve, sometimes quite dramatically. This is called the placebo response. The questions are: Why does this happen? Did the patients fake having pain at the beginning? How could a placebo cause so much improvement?

There are some answers to these puzzling questions from the world of research. The act of taking a pill and believing it might work is in itself a powerful psychological and biological intervention that can make pain genuinely better. In addition to this, neuroimaging research is showing us that when patients take a placebo medication and get better, they show the same changes in their brains as people who get better while taking actual medication. None of this research negates the fact that medications are effective (if they were not more effective than placebos, they would not receive Food and Drug Administration [FDA] approval. But the placebo response powerfully supports the role of belief and the complex interactions between psychology and biology in any effective treatment regimen. We should never mistakenly believe that because some patients responded to placebo that they never really had pain, or that all their pain was "all in their heads." Just remember, the brain is indeed in a person's head, and this brain, based on bio-psycho-social issues, can positively and negatively modulate our pain response.

62. Can I have a drink or two to help me cope with pain?

All three of the authors enjoy alcohol in moderation. We thought we should add this disclaimer so that you understand why we are very opposed to using alcohol to control pain. This opinion is not coming from a puritanical approach to alcohol consumption, but our strong opposition to alcohol use for pain management is based on a simple fact—it's a very bad idea for multiple reasons.

Alcohol use for pain management is a dead-end street. First, it is fairly ineffective as a pain "medicine," and what little effect it has wears off quickly. This often leads to increased use, which creates a whole new

Alcohol use for pain management is a dead-end street.

series of difficulties. You are advised to ignore the siren song of alcohol and instead seek other sources of help, both non-medication and medication types, for optimum pain management.

If you are already trapped in the vicious cycle of alcohol and chronic pain, we suggest you seek help from your medical professionals immediately. We as professionals have unfortunately far too often met people who have waited far longer than they should have to seek help. We urge you not to do so. Ask yourself today: Are you using alcohol excessively and inappropriately to control your chronic pain (or for any other reason, for that matter)? Is anyone around you—such as family members or friends—concerned about your use of alcohol? Are you getting into legal, occupational, or educational problems as result of your alcohol use? If the answer to any of these is "yes," immediate action is needed. Step one is to visit a trusted healthcare professional and report all that is happening. There are better ways of being helped than by misusing alcohol.

PART FOUR

Medications for Pain Treatment

What are the different types of pain medicines available to help me, and how do they work?

Are all antidepressants equally effective treatments for pain?

I heard that some patients taking pain medicine have developed tolerance, what is that, and how can I avoid it?

More . . .

63. What are the different types of pain medicines available to help me, and how do they work?

There is very good news to report in response to this question. There are now multiple medications, both approved and not approved by the Food and Drug Administration (FDA), that doctors have available to help you with your chronic pain.

There are literally dozens of classes of medications that have been demonstrated to help with pain, and each of these classes often has multiple medications in them (**Table 3**). Many of these medications are quite expensive, but a surprisingly large number are generic brands and are therefore affordable for almost everyone.

There are many over-the-counter (OTC) medications available in our stores; these usually include acetaminophen or one of the NSAIDs (non-steroidal anti-inflammatory drugs). These are effective and safe if used per directions on the bottle. Do remember, however, that just because a medication is available over-the-counter does not mean it is entirely safe! Protect these medications from children so that accidental overdoses do not occur. Also, these OTC medications sometimes can mix poorly with other medications, so your doctors should always know what OTC medications you are taking.

There also are many types of prescription medications. Many of them are in a class called opioids. These are reserved for acute pain and are to be used in chronic pain only when other options have been exhausted. We will discuss these medications in more detail in Question 67. There are also many medications in an antidepressant class that have demonstrated effectiveness in certain kinds of chronic pain disorders. And then there

Table 3 Commonly Used Medications for Pain Control
(Please note this is only a partial list. Check with your doctor if you have any questions.)

• Aspirin
• Acetaminophen

• Nonsteroidal Anti-Inflammatory Drugs (NSAIDs)
  ▪ ibuprofen
  ▪ naproxen
  ▪ fenoprofen
  ▪ ketoprofen
  ▪ indomethacin
  ▪ meloxicam
  ▪ diclofenac

• COX-2 Inhibitor   ▪ celecoxib

• Topical Medication (medications applied to the skin)
  ▪ lidocaine patches
  ▪ NSAID patches
  ▪ capsaicin cream

• Opioid Medications
  ▪ morphine
  ▪ hydrocodone
  ▪ meperidine
  ▪ methadone
  ▪ buprenorphine
  ▪ tramadol
  ▪ pentazocine
  ▪ codeine
  ▪ oxycodone

• Anticonvulsant Medications
  ▪ gabapentin
  ▪ pregabalin
  ▪ valproate
  ▪ carbamazepine

• Antidepressant Medications
  ▪ amityptyline
  ▪ duloxetine
  ▪ milnacipran

are medications that have effects on multiple brain chemicals, such as opioids and norepinephrine that can also be effective. Finally, there are multiple medications in a class called anti-epileptics that also have been demonstrated to be effective in some pain conditions.

Medications for Pain Treatment

The research world has taken notice of the fact that chronic pain conditions are still in need of better, safer, more effective medications. As a result, literally scores of medications are in various phases of clinical development, and hopefully in the near future will be available for use in clinics. We urge you to consult with your health care provider and agree on what medication(s) are most appropriate for your specific chronic pain condition.

64. I hear that some antidepressants can be helpful with pain but that does not make sense to me. How does that work and which kind of pain do they work for the best?

We understand why this might be confusing, but we think we can clear up the confusion. Many antidepressant medications work by modulating the body's levels of **serotonin** and **norepinephrine**. Serotonin and norepinephrine are names of brain chemicals that are used to transmit information from one cell to another. This information is carried electrically, but at the place where two nerves come together, the brain uses chemicals such as these to help information move forward. If you recall from reading our answers to the previous questions, these two brain chemicals play a significant role in pain control. There is significant evidence that in people with chronic pain, there are abnormalities in these two neurotransmitters.

Because the brain and the spinal column are rich in both of these two neurotransmitters—as well as the receptors on which they work—you can quite conceivably see why in many individuals with chronic pain, modulating serotonin and norepinephrine may be valuable.

Serotonin

A monoamine neurotransmitter (a chemical substance that the brain and the body use to help transmit information between nerves) involved with multiple bodily functions, including digestion, blood clotting, temperature, and mood and anxiety regulation.

Norepinephrine

A catecholamine (type of monoamine) synthesized from dopamine. Norepinephrine may act as a hormone, when secreted into the bloodstream from the adrenal medulla, or as a neurotransmitter in the central nervous system and sympathetic nervous system where it is released by noradrenergic nerve endings.

So, what are some of the medications available to you and your clinician to change the brain levels of these chemicals so that your pain problems are reduced? There are many medications that have previously been approved for the management of depression, but this takes nothing away from the fact that they may also, as a result of modulating serotonin and norepinephrine, be useful medications in pain management. One anti-depressant, called milnacipran, is approved for the treatment of fibromyalgia. Another antidepressant, duloxetine, is approved for three different pain conditions: fibromyalgia, diabetes related nerve pain, as well as chronic musculo-skeletal pain (like back pain or osteo-arthritis joint pain). And remember, these medications reduced pain even when depression was not present. This really does show that the word "antide-pressant" does not fully describe how many different things these medications, that work on multiple neurotransmitters, can accomplish.

The medications that are classically thought of as anti-depressants work for depression, depressed patients with pain, and patients with pain who do not have depression. Thus, we can see that these medications have multiple uses because of how they work (their mechanism of action) rather than how they are marketed.

These antidepressant medications are obviously helpful in chronic pain or depression states when only one of these conditions exist, but it can also be a "two for the price of one" deal when an individual has both depression and pain. So, the take home message might be: don't just judge a book by its cover; dig deeper, because there might be some wonderful benefits you can get by doing so! This has certainly proven to be the case with many antidepressants.

65. *Are all antidepressants equally effective treatments for pain?*

The short answer is no, but this question deserves a longer answer. This is what we know from preclinical (animal) studies of pain—norepinephrine is crucially important in chronic pain relief, and if serotonin modulation is present along with it, then perhaps the pain control is even better. Clinical human studies appear to support the idea that the presence of norepinephrine is crucial for an antidepressant to work as a good chronic pain medication. In fact, meta-analyses (when multiple studies are combined to increase the power of observation) show this trend too—it is the dual-mechanism medications, or the ones that work with both serotonin and norepinephrine, that work better than single-neurotransmitter antidepressants (usually it is serotonin only) for chronic pain.

Based on these fairly robust findings, most treatment guidelines and experts in the field of chronic pain recommend the more efficacious dual-action antidepressants over single-action antidepressants. The fortunate thing is that there are a number of older and newer dual-action antidepressants available, and it is best to work with your clinician to find which might be best for your specific situation.

We will share a concern here. Despite the fact that data convincingly show that dual-action antidepressants work better for chronic pain, we unfortunately far too often see pain patients being treated with single-action antidepressants. This is often a mistake, and patients end up getting inadequate benefits from the medication. We would urge you, the patient, to play an active role in discussing the choice of medication with your clinician. At the end of the day, the goal is to use the most efficacious medication with the least side-effect burden.

66. I understand that some medications are FDA-approved and some are not. What does this mean for my doctor and me?

To better understand this issue, let's first look at how medications are approved in our country. When a pharmaceutical company has a new medication that works in animal models, the company then approaches the FDA and gets approval for human trials. At this point, the FDA only allows research patients to get the medication. Once the pharmaceutical company has enough data on the safety and efficacy of the medication, they submit all the data to the FDA for potential approval. Only if the FDA then finds the medication safe and useful for general human use is it granted approval. At that point, it is sold in pharmacies and your doctor can prescribe it.

The thing to remember is that the FDA does not approve the medication only; it approves the medication for a specific condition or conditions. However, the law allows a clinician to prescribe any approved medication for any appropriate condition. So, if the medication is prescribed for a condition for which the FDA has not formally granted approval, this is then considered "off-label" prescribing. This is not necessarily bad, as often some of the most efficacious medications for a condition may not have FDA approval.

You may be wondering why a medication does not have all sorts of approval. This is because it is not possible for a pharmaceutical company to get approvals for all possible conditions. If a physician prescribes a mediation that is "on-label," that is ideal, but this option is not available for every situation. Sometimes a medication is available as a generic, and as there is little financial incentive to get new indications; a branded version of the same medication won't be subjected to the time and cost necessary to get an FDA indication. It costs millions of dollars to obtain a new indication for a medication. A physician, based on experience and/or clinical data, may think that even an off-label medication is appropriate for your needs and prescribe it for you. This is perfectly legal, and often the right thing to do. However, it is not always a good idea. In the history of medicine, using medications off-label has often proven to be useless, or worse, harmful. Therefore, if a medication is being prescribed to you, it is a good idea to ask your physician if it is FDA-approved for the use being prescribed. If it's not, we recommend that you have a discussion about why an off-label medication is still the right choice for you and what the positives and negatives may be from such a decision.

67. What are opioids, and what is their role in chronic pain management?

Opioid medications (also often called opiate, although opiates are strictly speaking chemicals that originate from poppy) are one of the greatest advances ever made in the history of pain management. **Opioids** have been used by mankind for many centuries for both good and bad reasons. These medications are derived from opium poppy plants, and their discovery, purification, and ultimate medicinal, high-quality preparations have been a boon to mankind. Their importance in pain management cannot be overstated.

Opioids

Medications and substances generated by our brain cells that attach themselves to receptors on the cell membranes, that specifically respond to them. Opioids are centuries-old medications, and if derived from a plant they are called natural, but they can also be semisynthetic or synthetic.

Before we talk about the many positives of this class of medications, it is also important to realize that opioids also have caused significant human suffering. Millions upon millions of people have become addicted to them or have died as a result of an overdose. Wars have been fought over them, and even today, Taliban militias in

Afghanistan derive their main source of income from the opium trade. That is why opium and medications derived from it have such an interesting role in our society.

All of us, whether we have chronic pain conditions or not, and even if we have never taken an opioid medication, have opioid receptors in our brain. In other words, we all naturally produce substances called enkephalines, dynorphins, and endorphins that alter our mood and pain threshold.

Many different types of opioid medications are available. Some of them are considered synthetic—in other words, they don't occur naturally, but were synthesized in a laboratory and are known to work on the opioid receptors in our brain. Different opioid medications have different potencies. This means that a milligram of one particular opioid medication may be stronger or weaker than a milligram of another opioid medication. Also, half-life, which is a measure of how long a medication stays in our system, is also different amongst medications. Finally, some opioids are considered full agonists of opioid receptors; that is, they only activate the opioid receptors in our system. Others are partial agonists, and some are full antagonists (i.e., these medications actually oppose the effects of opioid medications). Thus, you and your doctor need to know a lot about opioid medications before one is prescribed for you. Fortunately, most pain doctors are quite familiar with nearly all of these issues.

Another extremely important question to ask is when opioid medications should be used for chronic pain. You might be saying to yourself that these medications sound so bad that you should do anything you can to stay away from them. That would be incorrect thinking.

Medications for Pain Treatment

We believe, based on the enormous body of literature we have, that in chronic pain management, opioid medications should be used only when other medications appropriate for the condition have failed to be effective. However, it is equally important *not* to hold back from using opioids when they are indicated. The sad truth is that opioids are both overused and underused in our society. Many people who have no medical need for these medications use them and are harmed by them. By the same token, many patients who suffer from chronic pain who could benefit from such medications don't take them, as clinicians are sometimes overly afraid of prescribing them.

The challenge here is to understand when to consider the use of opioid medications. There is no one answer that fits all patients. However, we recommend keeping the following rule in mind: chronic pain not well managed by non-opioids is a signal to begin a conversation between patients and their clinicians about the positives and negatives of using an opioid medication. When they are needed, opioid medications can be hugely helpful, but their use should be monitored quite carefully, and the lowest effective dose for the shortest needed duration should be employed.

Chronic pain not well managed by non-opioids is a signal to begin a conversation between patients and their clinicians about the positives and negatives of using an opioid medication.

68. I have read in the newspapers about people dying from an overdose of pain medication. Is this true, and how can I prevent this from happening to me?

Sadly, this is true. Most often, the pain medications implicated are opioids. Occasionally, these overdoses occur in combination with other medications. Tragically, the individual who dies from combination medication overdose is often taking an excessive number of medications or has accidently taken too much medication. This is extremely unfortunate, and it often makes clinicians overly hesitant to prescribe opioid medications, even when their use is clinically indicated. Opioids in excessive doses can suppress breathing (particularly when combined with sleep medication or alcohol), sometimes leading to respiratory failure and death. Every emergency room has seen patients come in with overdoses. The trend now is for young college age kids to experiment with illegally diverted medications, with the result being that they slip into coma and occasionally die. Even if your medication becomes less effective, do *not* self-adjust your dose—this can lead to a lot of problems for you. Consult your clinician; he or she will appreciate such open communication.

Prevention is the key to avoiding dangerous overdoses. Don't ever use an opioid medication unless you and your clinician feel it is the best decision for you. Make sure your clinician knows about all other medications (over-the-counter, prescription, and herbal) you might be taking, as there are some dangerous drug interactions between certain medications and opioids. Take the medication only as prescribed. Opioids are actually safe medications if used the way we recommend (**Table 4**). As so much illegal opioid medication is diverted from patient to family or friends, *never* share your medication with anyone and store it properly so that it is not stolen. You have a responsibility to use this medication safely. Finally, if you notice side effects such as excessive sleepiness, unsteady gait, or foggy memory, be sure to let your clinician know, as this might alert him or her of the need to potentially lower your dose to prevent any difficulties.

Medications for Pain Treatment

Table 4   Steps to Take to Avoid Dangerous Overdoses

Only take opioids if prescribed for you.
Never "borrow" or use someone else's opioid medication.
Never "share" opioid medications with anyone.
Inform doctor about all other medications you are taking.
Take only as much, and as frequently as prescribed.
If you notice unusual side effects (e.g., excessive sleepiness, mental fogginess, trouble walking) report this to your doctor immediately.

69. I heard that some patients taking pain medicine have developed tolerance. What is that, and how can I avoid it?

Tolerance

A pharmacological phenomenon in which a person who takes a certain dose of medication on a regular basis notices a gradual decrease in benefits derived from the medication.

Let's first define **tolerance**. It is a pharmacological phenomenon in which a person who takes a certain dose of medication on a regular basis notices a gradual decrease in its benefits. This is a fairly common phenomenon, and it appears as if the body is finding a way to counter the medication. Tolerance is not always a bad thing—developing tolerance to side effects is actually a very positive development. What is not positive is when the tolerance develops to the positive effects of a medication, as this is quite frustrating to patients with chronic pain as well as to clinicians.

There is no foolproof way to prevent tolerance from developing; however, there are some strategies that can be effective to counter tolerance once it develops. First, tolerance does develop often, and if it does in your case, it is not your or your clinician's fault. Second, if your medication becomes less effective, let your clinician know. One way to counter tolerance is to increase the dose of the medication, assuming it is safe to do so.

Another way to counteract tolerance is to change your medication, and it is common to rotate pain medications for this reason. This appears to "fool" the body, and it is not uncommon to obtain relief from symptoms by such changing of medications.

70. Why do doctors sometimes combine medicines? Is it safe?

As you well know by now, chronic pain is created by amazingly complex and interconnected systems in our body. Different brain and body chemicals often control these different systems. When there is no pain, there is perfect harmony between these chemicals and all is well.

Multiple systems typically go haywire in the brains and bodies of people with chronic pain. Often, one single medication is able to correct the imbalance and the person will get relief from the chronic pain. However, in other cases this is not possible, and doctors must combine medications to bring relief to the individual. This fact reflects the body's complexity and how often chronic pain can be resistant to one medication alone.

Occasionally, doctors combine medications for another reason, not necessarily to help with pain, but to make a medication better tolerated by the patient. While this is not an ideal practice, one often has to resort to this technique in the quest for dominance over chronic pain.

Some medication combinations are very safe while others are problematic, and some are outright dangerous and potentially life-threatening. This is why we recommend that before you add any medication, be it over-the-counter or a prescription medication, inform your doctor and perhaps ask this question directly: "Do you know this combination to be safe?" This will alert your doctor to check for drug interactions and ensure safety. Remember, it is both your doctor's and your responsibility to have open lines of communication.

There are so many medications and potential beneficial and harmful combinations that it is impossible to give you a full list of these here. However, if medication combinations are done wisely and thoughtfully, they can be very helpful. Thus, don't fear medication combinations, but maintain safety by talking openly and communicating with your clinical team.

71. What are some of the side effects of opioid medications, and how can I manage them?

Opioid medications deserve our respect, both for the benefits they can deliver and for their side effects. The use of opiates always involves an assessment of a risk/benefit ratio that should be in the patient's favor. If the danger from opioids outweighs the benefits, they should not be used.

Opioids, like all other medications, can cause side effects some quite serious, and some less so. Knowing what these side effects are and how they can be managed empowers you. Some of the most serious side effects, typically in overdose situations, are breathing suppression, coma, and death. We discussed this issue in more detail in Question 67.

Constipation is another common, and often quite a significant problem with opioids. If constipation is mild there are a number of things you can do to combat it, such as increasing the amount of natural fiber in your diet, increasing your water intake, or eating a cup or a half-cup of high-fiber cereal (such as Fiber One™). Also make sure you are not eating too much cheese or peanut butter (two things we have found to cause constipation in some patients). If the constipation is more than mild, and you are having stomach pains or bloating, getting medical advice early is crucial so that you and your doctor can take immediate steps to prevent constipation from becoming a bigger problem.

Memory fogginess, mental slowing, and sleepiness are common side effects of opioids. Some ways to counter these problems are to inform your doctor if they occur so that he or she can reduce your opioid dose, change the time of the day you take your medications, or add other medications to counter these side effects. Please don't suffer needlessly; your clinician has a number of options to assist you with these side effects. Another side effect is slowed-motor reaction time, which can make driving dangerous. Be watchful, particularly early in treatment when you don't quite know how the medication is affecting you. Be aware that sometimes your motor reflexes can slow down, and mental fogginess can occur weeks, months, or even years after starting an opioid medication, so be on your guard. It is important to protect yourself and others.

There are more potential side effects of opioid medications but you and your clinician should discuss them in more detail during your visits. You shouldn't be overly scared of opioids—millions of people safely use opioid medications with a minimum of side effects. Keep working closely with your clinician, as this is the best way to get the most out of your medication with minimum difficulties.

72. Is it true that opioids can make my fibromyalgia worse?

This is actually a possibility for many patients with fibromyalgia (FM). As you know from reading other sections of this book, FM is a complex disorder involving a process called central sensitization that plays an important role in creating chronic pain. Opioid medications appear to be relatively ineffective in altering this. Additionally, recent research has shown that people with FM have lower numbers of opioid receptors in their brains. All this adds up to opioids not being the medications of choice for treatment in the early stages of FM. This fact has led to most worldwide treatment guidelines discouraging clinicians from utilizing opioids to treat FM. There is even more worrisome information—some patients with FM, if exposed to opioids for long periods of time, actually have an increase in pain. This is explained best by the complex pain mechanism of FM, as described above and elsewhere in this book. Thus, the take home message is that if you suffer from FM, try to avoid opioid medications. If you do end up taking them, consider taking them at the lowest dose for the shortest period of time possible. Scientific evidence strongly supports this recommendation.

73. My family tells me that no matter what, I should not take any medication with addictive potential. Are they giving me good advice?

This is not good advice. Your family members are probably only trying to protect you from the harmful effects of addictive medications. But what if you needed a medication for chronic pain that did have the potential to cause addiction? What if other non-addictive potential medications were not working for you? Would the rule of avoiding addictive medications at all costs still be in your best interests?

We think not. Unquestionably the addition of potentially addictive medications should be reserved for chronic pain use only when other medication and surgical/non-pharmacological options are not helping. But to live with chronic pain is a living nightmare for many people, and medications with addictive potential, when used wisely and carefully, can be hugely helpful. You have a right to be in as little pain as possible. Particularly with advances in pharmacotherapy, many opioid medications are becoming safer and more useful. You may try to avoid addicting medications, but if necessary, our recommendation is to avail yourself of such treatment options. The caveat, as always, is to do so under a clinician's guidance and keep the risk–benefit ratio of any medication firmly in mind.

74. How can epilepsy medications work for pain?

Epilepsy is a disorder of the brain in which electrical activity is disrupted to the point that a person suffers a seizure. There is a whole class of medications that work by acting on brain chemicals to suppress this aberrant brain electrical activity. These medications are generally called antiseizure medications. They generally work by either increasing the effects of inhibitory brain chemicals or by decreasing the effects of excitatory brain chemicals. As you should know quite well by now, chronic pain has a similar pathology. The pathology in chronic pain can occur at the level of nerves in the body, but even more so in the dorsal horn of the spinal column. In other words, in chronic pain, the pain-inhibitory system is weaker than it should be, and the excitatory system is stronger than it should be. Does it then not sound like these epilepsy medications would make a good choice for chronic pain?

Data show that they often are a good choice. Many different seizure medications have been studied, and quite a few have FDA indications for the treatment of chronic pain conditions. Thus, it may be wise to think of medications such as these in a much broader fashion. Yes, they can be very useful for chronic pain management. Note, however, that even though these medications fall in the large category of antiseizure medications, or anti-epilepsy medications, they are often very different in how they work. Therefore, a seizure medication may work for a certain kind of pain disorder but not others, or it may not be effective in pain management at all. Selecting the right medication for your particular needs is critically important. Also, some seizure medications have FDA approval, but most do not. Please discuss the implications of this with your clinician. Now, if your clinician recommends an antiseizure medication to you for chronic pain, you will understand the rationale behind it. As always, discuss the potential positive and negative consequences of this option fully with your clinician.

Many different seizure medications have been studied, and quite a few have FDA indications for the treatment of chronic pain conditions.

75. Is it true that a common side effect of pain medication is weight gain? How can I prevent this from happening to me?

It is true that some, but thankfully not all, medications for pain management can cause weight gain. We appreciate a discussion about this, because gaining weight, regardless of cause, is strongly associated with worsened physical and mental health. For you as a chronic pain sufferer, weight gain is even more problematic than it is for most people, as you may already be having trouble with mobility, and weight gain might make it worse.

Space limitations preclude us from being able to provide you with an exhaustive list of medications that can cause weight gain. Having said that, asking your clinician about the weight gain potential of any medication or medications you are taking is crucial. Preferably, you will have this conversation even before the medication is started. If this discussion did not happen at that time, it is never too late to discuss this. Remember: An ounce of prevention is worth more than a pound of treatment!

Being chronically in pain is often by itself a risk factor for weight gain. This is true for at least two reasons. First, people with chronic pain are often less mobile, which leads to lower calorie expenditure. Second, the body responds to chronic pain by altering its internal chemical and hormonal milieu, and this can result in weight gain. As to why some medications cause weight gain, this too is because of multiple mechanisms. However, the most common reason that medications cause weight gain is that they make people more hungry, so more calories are ingested.

We recommend the following concrete steps for you. Ask your clinician about potential side effects before starting any medication (or as soon as possible after), and ask specifically about weight gain as an issue. We know from our experience as clinicians and from the scientific literature that it is extremely important to counteract the potential risk for weight gain by taking two steps as soon as you can. These two steps are: (1)

gradually increase exercise time, intensity, and frequency (this topic is discussed in Question 65), and (2) make changes to your nutrition. Our experience and data support the real validity of these two interventions. They will either prevent weight gain or limit it. If your doctor is able to recommend another medication that is equally effective but has less weight gain potential, by all means discuss changing to it. Often joining a support group such as Weight Watchers or joining a structured exercise program such as Curves can be helpful. We have had patients who have taken advantage of such interventions, and they are testimonials to their effectiveness. You don't necessarily need to join such organizations if you feel that you are self-motivated and you can get the job done. But if you can't do it by yourself, there is absolutely no shame in asking your clinician, family, friends, or organizations for extra help. Remember, controlling weight is a lifelong project, but it does not have to be lifelong torture. Changing habits gradually leads to permanent lifestyle changes and will help you mange your weight for a lifetime.

76. Do regular over-the-counter pain medications help? How safe are they?

Over-the-counter pain medications are used millions of times each year, and most of the time they are helpful and safe. However, it would be an error to assume that just because they are OTC, you do not need to exercise some caution in using them. Used as directed, they are quite safe, but they can do significant harm if inappropriately used. For example, acetaminophen (in medications like Tylenol and dozens of other OTC medications) is very often a cause of life-threatening overdose, both intentional and accidental. Taking too much acetaminophen can so badly damage the liver

Over-the-counter pain medications are used millions of times each year, and most of the time they are helpful and safe. However, it would be an error to assume that just because they are OTC, you do not need to exercise some caution in using them.

that it is one of the leading causes of liver failure and liver transplants.

You should also be aware that most OTC medications have been better studied for acute pain for which the medications were taken for relatively short periods of time. Much less is known about the safety of these medications when used for longer periods. Keep the rule we have often discussed, firmly in mind: all medications, even OTC medications, should be used at the lowest dose for the shortest length of time. If they are indeed needed long-term, it is best to be under the watchful eye of your clinician. Over-the-counter medications are quite safe, but not entirely so. Use them as directed by your clinician, and exercise caution.

77. Once I start a medication, will I have to take it for the rest of my life?

This is a difficult question to answer, because chronic pain situations differ. What is really at stake with this question, however, is this: What if you were to get substantial benefit from a medication that went away when you stopped the medication? Would you want to stop an effective, well-tolerated medication and go back to having pain, or would you be willing to continue taking the medication indefinitely?

The complexities of treating chronic pain make this dilemma all too real for many patients, because often a medication might be indicated for long periods of time—perhaps life. This is not an "I have to take the medication" situation, but rather an "I choose to take the medication" situation. However, with professional help, one can in most instances detoxify from addicting medications such as opiates and benzodiazepines. We will not say that detoxing is as easy as a walk in the park, but modern advances in detoxification techniques have made the process much more comfortable and successful. When you do have to choose medications with addicting potential, the goal is to use the smallest dose for the shortest amount of time. This last statement is true for most patients, although some patients on chronic therapy with potentially addictive medications may have to take them for the rest of their lives because their pain is too much to bear without them. These patients have made a choice to stay on medications for life, and we support their well-thought out, informed decision. As every situation is different, you should pose this question to your clinician, too. It is a difficult, complex question, and everyone's needs are different. We hope that you use these medications for short amounts of time, but if you need them for a longer period of time, as long as it is well thought out with a full understanding of the risks and benefits, we support that decision entirely.

Sue said:

"I choose to take the medication" leaves me in the driver's seat and not a passive participant. I'm a Type I diabetic and issues around food are similar to this question about medication. Tell me I can't have certain food (taking the decision away from me), and I'm likely to eat it anyway. It's all about being an active participant. I believe this is true when it comes to decisions about taking medications.

78. What role, if any, does marijuana play in pain management?

This is a hugely controversial topic that our society is currently grappling with. No clear resolution appears to be on the horizon. Some states in our country have liberal laws regarding the use of marijuana for medical purposes, while other states are restrictive and only see such use of marijuana as a criminal offense.

Let's take a quick look at the scientific literature on this topic. Animal data actually do show that marijuana has activity against pain perception. There is significant research being conducted at this time to see if scientists can purify the active substances that give this pain relief, and also develop other medications that directly act on specific marijuana receptors in our brain. This knowledge does need to be counterbalanced with the knowledge that marijuana in many individuals has potential for addiction and problematic changes in behavior, motivation, concentration, drive, and sometimes mood.

The use of medicinal marijuana is so differently restricted in different states that you truly do need to consult your clinician for advice. Marijuana should never be a first-line choice for pain management. There are too many concerns regarding its use, as well as numerous unanswered questions. However, if multiple pain interventions have failed you, your state laws permit such use, and your clinician is well versed in the use of marijuana, it may be time to at least consider this as a treatment modality. Needless to say, the use of marijuana for pain management requires close self-monitoring by you and your clinical team.

Sue said:

The risks associated with medical marijuana seem similar to those associated with traditional pain medications (addiction potential, problematic changes in behavior, motivation, concentration, drive and sometimes mood). I've tried to avoid pain medications for those very reasons. The truth is no medication is without some risk. I like your suggestion of being fully informed of the risks and benefits.

79. What are non-steroidal anti-inflammatory drugs (NSAIDs) and COX-2 inhibitors and how do they work? Do they have any potential problems that I should know about?

These are some of the most widely used pain medications in the world, and as such are available in every country. Millions upon millions of people have taken them for one reason or another. Some common examples of **NSAIDs** include Advil and Naprosyn. The COX-2 inhibitor class of medications at one time had many members, but many of these have been withdrawn from the market. The best known COX-2 inhibitor still on the market is Celebrex. NSAIDs and **COX-2 inhibitors** work through a complex series of steps in our body, but ultimately they reduce the levels of chemicals that are pain-provoking. NSAIDs work by blocking the enzyme cyclooxygenase (COX). NSAIDs block both forms of COX, known as COX-1 and COX-2. They reduce inflammation, which is in itself a pain-generator. There are multiple types of NSAIDs that are available OTC and some that are available only by prescription from a clinician. COX-2 inhibitors are a subtype of NSAIDs that are more specific by working only on the COX-2 pathway. Because they spare the COX-1 pathway, they have fewer gastrointestinal and other side effects.

Many people use these medications for a short period of time, for an occasional headache, for a few days for painful menstrual periods, a sprained ankle, and so forth. There appear to be minimal concerns when these medications are used for short periods, as long as the person is healthy and does not have any stomach ulcers, gastrointestinal bleeding, blood-clotting difficulties, or cardiovascular problems.

NSAIDs

Abbreviation designating nonsteroidal anti-inflammatory drugs; medications with analgesic (pain-reducing) and antipyretic (fever-reducing) properties. Higher doses also have anti-inflammatory activity (reducing inflammation).

COX-2 inhibitors

Medications designed to inhibit cyclooxygenase-2, an enzyme involved in the synthesis of prostaglandins. These agents have anti-inflammatory and analgesic (painkiller) properties.

The real worry centers on the use of these medications in long-term situations. By long-term we mean any length of time longer than a couple of weeks. Some people take these medications for years. With one particular COX-2 inhibitor, Vioxx, there was so much concern about increased cardiovascular death rates that the medication was withdrawn. Hundreds of lawsuits against the manufacturer of this medication are still pending. The problem for clinicians and patients is that COX-2 inhibitor medications often are so effective that stopping them becomes a real challenge. Although real, the risk for cardiac problems is fairly small, so this risk needs to be balanced against the very real daily benefits many patients receive from these medications.

The NSAIDs are fairly well-tolerated and, in our experience, few patients develop significant side effects if these medications are used for a short time. It's best not to take them on an empty stomach, as some patients do report nausea in this situation. Long-term use does carry some risks, particularly bleeding of the stomach or other areas of the gastrointestinal tract. This is why if you already have such a problem, or are at a high risk of developing it, doctors will not recommend this class of medication. Sometimes they will recommend preventative treatment with a medication to reduce stomach acids so that these NSAIDs will not cause stomach bleeding.

COX-2 medications were invented for precisely this very concern with "older" NSAIDs. The thought was that a medication with activity at just the COX-2 enzyme would reduce the risk of gastrointestinal bleeding, because this happens through the COX-1 enzyme inhibition. And this indeed has proven to be true. This is why, when these medications were released in the market, they were hailed as a great success. However, the emergence of subsequent information indicating a significant increase in cardiovascular deaths led to much less use of these medications. COX-2 inhibitors are still available in the United States, but as mentioned above, you and your doctor should carefully weigh the risks and benefits of these medications for your particular situation, particularly if long-term use is considered, before making a decision.

80. Do steroids ever have a role in pain management?

Steroids are medications that can be lifesaving in many situations. They certainly do have a role in chronic pain, but their role is fairly limited because of the multiple side effects and potential dangers that accompany their use. When we talk about steroids, we are not referring to anabolic steroids, such as professional athletes abuse! Rather, we mean **corticosteroids**, which are part of the body's stress management system. As you know, sometimes chronic pain results from an inflammatory condition, such as rheumatoid arthritis. Quite often orthopedic surgeons or rheumatologists will inject a painful joint (whether because of osteoarthritis or a condition like rheumatoid arthritis) with corticosteroids. This can be quite helpful. Sometimes clinicians will also use oral tablets of steroids in order to control inflammation and to reduce pain. Sometimes pain doctors will inject a small amount of these steroids near the spinal column to reduce pain.

You do need to know this: while steroids can be very helpful medications, they can have substantial side effects, which limit their use quite significantly. Some of the side effects include weight gain, sleep disturbances, worsening mood, irritability, occasionally precipitating manic

Steroids

Both natural and synthetic chemicals that have different effects on the body. Natural steroids are essential for healthy living, and too much or too little can cause major problems. Steroids help people deal with stress and modulate inflammation and immune responses. Chronic pain disorders are often associated with irregular steroid activity.

Corticosteroids

A group of steroid hormones produced by the cortex of the adrenal gland or made synthetically. These "stress" hormones typically have anti-inflammatory and immunosuppressant properties.

episodes, electrolyte imbalances, weakening muscles, and an increased risk for diabetes. All doctors learn to both love and fear steroid medications for these reasons. We don't want to imply that steroid use is bad. On the contrary, the use of steroids for short periods of time (at least in most patients) can be a very wise move and sometimes a lifesaver. However, if steroids are to be used long-term, a very careful discussion of the risks and benefits should occur between the clinician, patient, and family. Clinicians who prescribe steroids do well to keep this rule in mind: use the smallest dose for the shortest amount of time, and carefully watch for any possible side effects. In conclusion, if you have to use steroids, definitely use them, but if you have alternatives, you may want to avail yourself of these other options to avoid or minimize steroid use. We recommend that you have this open conversation with your clinician about the pros and cons of using steroids in your particular situation.

PART FIVE

Interventional and Surgical Means of Treating Pain

Could surgery possibly help my chronic pain? If so, what kind of pain is most likely to respond to a surgical intervention?

What are the different kinds of surgeries that can help with chronic pain, and which doctors should I consult?

What are nerve blocks, and could they help me?

More . . .

81. Could surgery possibly help my chronic pain? If so, what kind of pain is most likely to respond to a surgical intervention?

Surgery is a definite option for many kinds of chronic pain. This is the good news. The bad news is that for many other kinds of chronic pain, surgery is no help at all. Let's talk more about this.

The type of chronic pain most responsive to surgery is nociceptive pain.

The type of chronic pain most responsive to surgery is nociceptive pain. This is pain that is clearly being generated from a specific organ or location. An example of this may be a hip joint that is very painful because of arthritic changes. In this case, a hip replacement typically gets rid of the pain entirely. Other types of chronic pain disorders, including neuropathic pain (pain because of diseased nerves, rather than an actual organ) or mixed pain disorders (pain because of abnormal pain processing) are not responsive to surgery.

The kind of pain you have plays a very large role in answering the question of whether surgery is an option for you. The other good news is that many conditions previously thought not to be candidates for surgical relief now are. Good examples come from the orthopedic world where joint replacements are available for multiple joints in your body. The quality of life improvement that this can deliver is amazing. Similarly, people suffering from chronic pain because of blood supply problems (such as partial occlusion of blood vessels) can also get a lot of relief from surgical correction.

A word of caution here is important: we have met chronic pain patients on whom surgery was repeatedly done even when they were not good candidates for it. This is not only expensive, but it can create more problems than solutions for some patients. Our advice, therefore, is to definitely ask your clinician if surgery is an option for relief of your chronic pain, but make your decision carefully, deliberately, and perhaps by even seeking a second opinion. The right kind of surgery in the right kind of patient can profoundly improve chronic pain. But wisdom and good judgment on the part of the patient and doctor are needed to achieve optimum outcomes. And if surgery is indeed strongly recommended and appropriate, we strongly urge you to consider this as an option for yourself. We can testify to surgery's enormous positive impact on patient lives when it is chosen wisely as an option.

82. What are the different kinds of surgeries that can help with chronic pain, and which doctors should I consult?

There are multiple kinds of surgeries with a good track record of helping people with chronic pain. And to offer you even better news, nearly every surgical specialty now has specific interventions to help with such pain conditions. We will give you a few examples. The list of surgical options we are discussing here is not comprehensive because of space limitations, but know that every surgical specialty is acutely aware of the plight of patients with chronic pain and has a number of options to offer you. Just remember the caveat we offered in the last question. While a number of chronic pain sufferers can be helped with surgery, many cannot, and they should not get unnecessary surgery. Discuss these issues carefully with your clinician.

Let's take a look at some specialties and what they can do to help you. Orthopedic surgeons can replace your joints, repair your ligament tears, or often fix other surgically repairable parts of your joints and bones. They can help back pain patients by creating bigger outlets for nerves that are being compressed by bones in the spinal column, as well as removing bulging discs that are pressing upon nerves. They can remove tumors and blood clots that can cause pain. Neurosurgeons can also remove tumors, blood clots, or ruptured discs. Gynecologists can remove adhesions, tumors, or other reasons for pain in female patients. Urologists can do similar things in the entire urinary system. Similarly, cardiovascular surgeons can unblock blood vessels when they are a cause of chronic pain. This list goes on and on.

With regard to which doctor to consult, we suggest starting with your primary care physician whom you trust and know to be up to date on the recent developments. He or she can serve as a triage person to guide you to the right specialties. Often, more than one specialty will need to get involved in your care. Because of this, to ensure that your care does not become fragmented, it is best to use the help of your primary care physician to ensure your surgical consults and procedures are well coordinated.

Sue said:

I have had three surgeries—the first two were successful, but the final surgery was only partially successful. I have limited range of motion and certain movements result in significant pain. I debated on having another surgery but decided I can manage my current situation with other interventions. However, if my situation changes and surgery is needed, I'm glad to know that's an option.

Nerve blocks

Injection of local anesthetic in the vicinity of nerves for temporary control of pain.

83. What are nerve blocks, and could they help me?

Nerve blocks are a significant new development in chronic pain management. To fully understand what nerve blocks are, let's quickly review the pain circuitry. If you recall, pain perception is accomplished by the body using a pain circuit that starts from an organ that includes nerves that carry pain signals up the spinal column to the brain, along with nerves that feed back from the brain, down the spinal column, to the organ. This is the pain circuit. Pain cannot be perceived by the brain if the nerve fibers carrying the electrical signals up to it are blocked. This is, in a nutshell, the science behind why, in some chronic pain patients, nerve blocks can be an option.

When a nerve block is done, the clinician identifies the nerve or nerve ganglion that is part of the pain circuit from where the chronic pain is originating. Then, under a careful surgical technique, a needle is inserted near this nerve or ganglion, and a local anesthetic or steroid is injected. When successful, this makes the nerve fire less often and become less effective in carrying pain signals to the spinal column. Nerve blocks only work if there is a specific nerve identified that is involved in your pain. For some pain disorders, this is very easy to do, and with other pain disorders it is essentially impossible. Nerve block medications are broadly categorized into two categories—ones that work for a few days or longer and those that are designed to permanently destroy a few nerves so that abnormal pain is blocked permanently in that pain circuit. This is called nerve ablation. Doctors in many types of specialties conduct nerve blocks to help chronic pain patents, but most often they are pain specialists with training in anesthesiology, or they are neurosurgeons. Ensure that you are a suitable candidate for nerve blocks and that your primary care physician recommends the specialist you see for a nerve block evaluation. Sometimes, nerve blocks are also done as part of a diagnostic procedure; that is, not really to gain sustained pain relief, but to allow the physician to discover whether a particular nerve or ganglion is involved in the pain problem.

As you can see, technology is marching ahead and helping more chronic pain sufferers. But, like any emerging technology, not all important questions regarding the use of nerve blocks have yet been answered. Thus, consult with your clinical team as you consider nerve blocks either for diagnostic or therapeutic purposes.

84. I have heard of people using an implanted medication pump that delivers pain medicines directly into the spinal column for pain control. This sounds very far-fetched, is this even true?

It is true! Medical technology has advanced to the point that, for certain kinds of chronic pain disorders in which other treatment options have failed; implanted pumps that deliver pain medications directly into the spinal column are available. This is how it works: a spinal surgeon implants a small tube into your spinal column, and a pump with a pain medication stored inside it is implanted elsewhere in the body. This technology is called **intrathecal pump therapy**. This sounds far-fetched, but it is an effective treatment as long as patient selection for this procedure is done carefully and thoughtfully.

Intrathecal pump therapy

Treatment based on the delivery of pain medication directly into the cerebrospinal fluid via a small medical device.

Who might be a candidate for this type of therapy? Based on our experience and reading of the literature, here is a short list of people with chronic pain who might benefit: patients with failed back surgery syndrome, patients with cancer pain, patients with reflex sympathetic dystrophy, and patients with painful cerebral palsy.

This is an expensive procedure, so expect some delay as your insurance company and doctor work out the logistics. Once you start considering this procedure, it is very important that you shop around for a well-known surgeon with expertise in this area before you settle on your final choice. If this is indeed the right fit for you, we encourage you to explore this option fully. This new technology does prove that a wide range of people from very different professional backgrounds (pain doctors, surgeons, engineers, etc.) are all working together to create innovative treatment options for chronic pain sufferers. We fully expect this collaboration to produce even more fruitful results as time goes by, so stay informed on its progress!

85. I saw Jerry Lewis talk on TV about an implanted pain-controlling nerve stimulator for his chronic back pain. What is that?

Jerry Lewis does suffer from chronic low back pain and has been a great spokesperson for the cause of chronic pain treatment. The device you ask about is another excellent advance in chronic pain management. These devices are called spinal cord stimulators, and they consist of electrodes that are thin wires that a surgeon implants into your spinal cord and an electrical generator, which is inserted under your skin. These two are connected, and the generator creates very tiny electrical impulses that travel up the electrodes to deliver these impulses to the nerves of your spinal column. As you already know by now, pain circuits function through the use of chemical and electrical signals. When the pain stimulator is delivering its charge, pain perception is diminished. Interestingly, creating these impulses from the outside makes our nerves less likely to fire inappropriately in ways that create chronic pain.

Thus, there is a sound medical logic in this approach to treating chronic pain. It sounds like science fiction, but it is actually a proven technology. Once the device is implanted and you have healed from the surgery, you and your doctor will work on adjusting the level of activity from the electrical stimulator. This is done in order to custom-fit your generator's output to your needs. Patients do not find the electrical activity from the generator painful, as the level of electrical impulse is very low—nothing like what comes out of the socket!

Again, careful selection of patients is crucial, as this is not for every kind of pain disorder. Most often, we have seen it being used in chronic back pain patients when other treatments have failed or worked only partially. It is expensive, to be sure, but it can be quite effective. Our review of the literature shows that about 50% to 75% of patients appear to derive benefit from it. Complication rates are fairly low, but not inconsequential. As always, if you think this type of stimulator might benefit you, discuss it with your doctor carefully, look into it yourself, and if it is appropriate for you, we encourage considering this option.

86. Is surgery a better treatment for pain than medications?

The simple answer to your question is that it depends on the situation. For some pain disorders, the answer to your question is not either this or that, but both. There are certain chronic pain disorders in which initial treatment is best accomplished with medications, and surgery only becomes a preferable option if medicines don't work sufficiently or if the condition worsens over time to the point that medications are no longer able to control the pain.

There are many other chronic pain disorders where surgery simply is not an option. This may be because the origin of pain is so diffuse that there is no surgery that can fix it, such as fibromyalgia. In these situations, one has to turn to non-surgical techniques to help control the pain. On the flip side, it would be a travesty of justice to not offer surgery to certain patients with chronic pain disorder, for example, in conditions such as joint replacements, removal of tumors that are causing pain, and so forth.

Because each chronic pain disorder is so different from every other one, and each patient's situation is quite different from anyone else's, we cannot specifically tell you if you need surgical or non-surgical treatment (or both) based solely on your diagnosis. However, you should partner with your medical team and ask them this question quite directly: "For my chronic pain, do we need to approach this non-surgically, surgically, or do we need to consider both?" Such a question will get the conversation started. Feel free to ask for more information, be it reading materials, Internet sites, or support groups. Surgery is not a benign, no-risk condition, and therefore the benefit–risk ratio needs to be balanced carefully as you make your decision. Finally, as a strong word of encouragement to you as a chronic pain sufferer, literally every month there are advances being made in both surgical and non-surgical treatments for pain.

Because each chronic pain disorder is so different from every other one, and each patient's situation is quite different from anyone else's, we cannot specifically tell you if you need surgical or non-surgical treatment (or both) based solely on your diagnosis.

87. I have had back pain for a long time— would imaging studies help my doctors properly diagnose it?

Did you know that back pain is one of the most common and one of the most expensive pain disorders? We sympathize with you and acknowledge the suffering you must have endured in terms of pain, limitations in functioning, and perhaps in financial losses. We will do our best to address this specific question regarding imaging studies fully.

First, let's establish the following fact: chronic back pain can occur from a large variety of causes. In any given person, the chronic pain could be originating from bones, muscles, ligaments, nerves, disc problems, or psychogenic reasons. With chronic back pain, it is actually mandatory to obtain (if it has not been obtained before) some kind of imaging study as part of the workup. Imaging studies include a large number of techniques such as X-rays, computed tomography (CT) scans, magnetic resonance imaging (MRI) scans, and sometimes even more specialized imaging techniques in which special dyes are injected in order to see anatomic details more clearly.

A number of potential causes of pain can be detected by one of the imaging techniques described in the last paragraph. Depending on the technique, one could see evidence of arthritis, disc bulging or a ruptured disc, a tumor, a curved spine (scoliosis), and so forth. Imaging is particularly needed if your chronic pain has significantly changed by either getting worse or by the type of pain. Additionally, if you have **radiating pain**—pain that shoots down your legs or your buttocks—it is quite important to obtain an imaging test that is most appropriate for your situation. The reason for this is that such a shooting pain often means there is nerve compression in your back, and speed in diagnosing and treating it is mandatory for you to achieve the best outcome possible.

Radiating pain

Pain felt in parts of the body where there is no cause of pain. Often caused by a "pinched," squeezed, or damaged nerve elsewhere. For example, a person can feel pain that shoots down the legs or buttocks even when the damage is in the pelvic region.

PART SIX

Coping With, Living With, and Thriving Despite Pain

What advice do you have for me if I would like to join a support group to connect with other people suffering from pain?

What are some coping skills that can help me and my family deal better with chronic pain?

Can complementary therapies or alternative therapies be helpful in pain management?

More . . .

88. What advice do you have for me if I would like to join a support group to connect with other people suffering from pain?

This is what we say—go for it! Your desire to get support makes sense at a number of levels. Humans are intensely social creatures, and when we are in chronic pain, quite inadvertently, we may actually become less social. This might reflect the fact that chronic pain makes you less mobile so you are out and about less, that because of time away from work you are not as much in contact with coworkers, or that because of stress or depression you just don't feel like being around other people. We have often seen these issues in chronic pain sufferers, and they are always unhelpful, and actually quite harmful to their well-being in the long-term. New research shows that the quality and quantity of human interaction has a direct bearing on our brains and mental health. Thus, whether we are suffering from pain or not, socializing is enormously important. Studies show that if socializing with others puts us in a more emotionally positive frame of mind, this will actually reduce how intensely our brains feel physical pain.

Support groups are a great way to accomplish exactly the type of social support that is so helpful. On top of this, a good support group will give you advice, support, needed direction, hope, encouragement, a sense of camaraderie, and a sense of being fully understood. This can be valuable beyond belief.

Because of the advances in technology, many support groups now occur over the Internet. You may want to explore whether one of these groups might be of benefit for you; however, there is still enormous value in face-to-face meetings, so you shouldn't ignore or avoid such "live" support groups. You can find such groups by asking your clinicians, as they most likely have other patients in local support groups, or by checking the local listings, with your pastor, or with religious leaders. Local newspapers often have wonderful lists of local support groups as part of their public service mission. And finally, if there is no support group to your liking, start one! The act of helping others is a powerful means of helping ourselves—this is one of the reason support groups are so helpful to one and all.

Many of our patients are helped by support groups. We, however, do want to offer you a small word of advice. Not all the information you get at support groups is necessarily true or helpful, and not all members are going to be of help to you. Some may actually criticize you or belittle your choices. Some of our patients have occasionally had such negative experiences in support groups. This is rare, but you need to be aware of this risk, and if you get advice or information you are unclear about, please check it out with your trusted clinician's help.

89. Is it realistic to expect 100% pain relief 100% of the time? If not, what should I realistically expect?

While we wish 100% of patients with chronic pain experienced 100% pain relief, this is not achievable given the limitations of the current state of our medical knowledge. The goal is a worthy one, and the right one, and one day perhaps we will achieve it. But being realistic is quite important; otherwise disenfranchisement with helping professionals can develop, which ultimately harms you. So, let's discuss this topic honestly and realistically, while maintaining a sense of optimism regarding your situation.

The truth about the state of pain management is that quite dramatic and positive developments have occurred in this field over the last 10 to 20 years.

The truth about the state of pain management is that quite dramatic and positive developments have occurred in this field over the last 10 to 20 years. This has happened with medications, psychotherapies, complementary medicine techniques, and surgical techniques. There are thousands of Americans who because of these techniques are now living lives essentially free of pain. But these thousands of individuals are outnumbered by millions of others who are better, but not cured of chronic pain. No clinician will ever treat you with the desire to help you gain anything less than 100% improvement, and if the technology or therapies exist to accomplish this goal for you, we are very glad for you. But if such technology or interventions are not available, then you are most likely not going to have the "100% fix." While this will undeniably disappoint you, don't let "perfect be the enemy of the good" and don't begin to believe that you can't be helped. Perhaps one day soon, your and your clinician's efforts will win out over the pain completely. Keep such hope; it is important that you have this lofty goal. But in the meantime, don't become disappointed if your goals are not immediately fulfilled.

What you should realistically expect truly depends on the cause of your chronic pain. You should expect improvement in most situations where you are doing all the things recommended for your specific situation. We hope over time success builds on success. Expect to work at it and to expend significant effort as you attempt to conquer chronic pain. We expect this will pay off handsomely for you in the long run.

90. How can I get my family and friends to fully understand my pain and how it affects me?

Implied in this question is the expression of a basic human need—that when we are hurting (figuratively or literally), we have a need to be understood and supported by our nearest and dearest. The need to have your family members understand your unfortunate chronic pain condition is very normal.

There are multiple reasons and issues that explain why your family might not fully understand your situation or be able to fully empathize. One might be as simple as that you or your clinicians may not have told them very much about your chronic pain condition. This could result from you being embarrassed about your pain condition and having minimized it. Talk directly to your family, offer them reading materials, perhaps take them with you to appointments with your healthcare providers, let them know about your suffering, and finally—and most importantly—*directly* communicate with them about how chronic pain is impacting you and what kind of emotional support you need from them. In many situations, such an approach works and the positive benefits that result can be tremendous. We all like our burdens shared. This is a basic human need.

It may be helpful for you to appreciate the fact that unless someone has walked in your shoes before, they most likely will have a hard time appreciating the amazingly powerful effect chronic pain can have on human life. This is not to make an excuse for your family or friends not offering you the support you deserve. On the contrary, approaching them with this premise in mind might help you structure your conversation with them in such a way that you don't come across as demanding, needy, or blaming. This approach may be particularly valuable with chronic pain disorders that are not immediately obvious to others because there are no obvious external signs of damage.

Coping With, Living With, and Thriving Despite Pain

Examples of such conditions include fibromyalgia, chronic headaches, and some kinds of neuropathic pain. If you had a cut or an open wound, outsiders' eyes immediately see a reason for you to be in pain. That's why the risk of not obtaining appropriate understanding and sympathy from others is enhanced in pain conditions that lack an obvious pain source.

No matter what your pain condition is, you deserve all the help, encouragement, and support from your family and friends that you can get. That is an unequivocal statement. Obtaining this might require patience and tact on your part. They may need to be better educated about your pain disorder, visit with your clinical team, or go to a support group with you. But no matter what means are used, we want you to have their support. We encourage you to seek this in such a way that you maximize your chances of obtaining it!

91. Should my doctors and I only focus on pain, or is it important to address my other difficulties, such as sleep, memory problems, and fatigue?

The answer to this question, unequivocally, is the following: all symptoms that impair you and your life as you live with chronic pain are targets of treatment. This advice we offer you without any reservations or hesitation.

Let's go over some background information as to why we so encourage treating all your symptoms. The three things you mention—sleep difficulties, memory problems, and fatigue—just by themselves cause significant impairment and problems in our lives. That in itself is enough reason to treat these issues through whatever means necessary. But our advice is even more meaningful if you appreciate all the research showing that sleep, fatigue, and memory problems all make pain outcomes much worse than they would be otherwise. Patients with these additional symptoms (and many patients with pain have them) have a harder time getting better, a lower rate of full recovery and a longer, tougher course in life. Despite their importance, clinicians often make the mistake of focusing just on pain and inadvertently forgetting to treat the associated difficulties. When this happens outcomes are always suboptimal.

What can be done to improve matters? First, appreciate that chronic pain rarely exists by itself. Sleep difficulties, memory difficulties, and fatigue tend to be common co-occurring conditions. Second, don't be silent about your issues, should they be present. Let your clinician team know, request that they help you not just with pain, but with all the symptoms that are bothering you. Fortunately, many treatments for pain can help more than pain symptoms. For example, certain medications are able to offer help for both pain and sleep relief. Often, however, one intervention is not able to address all your needs and you and your clinician will have to discuss together which combination of non-medication and medication treatments you should consider. The goal is, quite simply, to optimally control chronic pain and any other co-occurring condition. We may not be 100% successful 100% of the time, but that does not change the goals we have set for ourselves.

Finally, follow this advice. Do your best to track all your symptoms: chronic pain and whatever else is present along with it. We are on solid clinical and scientific ground when we say that doing so is in your best long-term and short-term interest.

92. Should I fight this pain by myself, or create a support system of family, friends, and medical professionals to deal with it?

Having read our responses to your questions so far, you probably can guess what our response to this question will be. There is absolute agreement between the authors that creating a team to help you deal with chronic pain is the right thing to do. But why this recommendation? You deserve to delve into this issue more thoroughly.

Humans are social creatures who do best in groups. This is in our genetic code; it is intertwined in our DNA. Our optimum mental and physical well-being occurs in group settings—in family units, marital units, extended family situations, our work environment, and our religious and social environments. Outstanding research published recently (Fowler JH, Christakis NA. BMJ) by social scientists reveals that our happiness, or lack thereof, is powerfully influenced by the level of happiness (or sadness) of those around us. Chronic pain by its very nature is a difficult situation for anyone to deal with. It is a burden, it is demoralizing, and it often drives us into isolation. It is a tough state of existence.

This, then, is the very reason to seek and create a highly supportive environment for yourself. Besides the fact that the support of others obviously helps you with tangible things, such as activities of daily living with which you might be having trouble, or with other issues, such as transportation, financial or occupational difficulties, we derive a lot of emotional strength from others, and this is at least as important as any practicality. And yes, healthcare providers are here for you not just to obtain chronic pain therapies, but also to offer you emotional support. This will improve the quality of your life, but just as importantly, it will increase the management of chronic pain.

Let's also appreciate this fact, startling as it may be: social isolation is far more than just a social state of being. It is also a powerful negative influencer of psychological and biological health. People who are isolated are at higher risk for developing stress-related disorders such as depression and anxiety. They are also more likely to have more infections as a result of weakened and improperly functioning immune systems. These are, of course, issues of importance to all, but for those with chronic pain who are already at higher risk for developing the difficulties we have just outlined, being socially isolated is even more problematic. Thus, we strongly urge you to obtain support for as wide a circle of people that you can while you deal with and fight to overcome your pain disorder.

93. I sometimes feel guilty, embarrassed, and ashamed of my chronic pain, as it limits my ability to function. What advice can you offer me to help deal with this?

It is often the case to feel the emotions described here. Needless to say, you have no reason to feel embarrassed or ashamed, as you are, in many ways, a victim of the chronic pain you endure and deserve sympathy and support from all, but particularly from yourself. So, why then, do some people with chronic pain feel these negative emotions of embarrassment and shame?

The answer to this is complex, but deserves a full discussion. Part of the answer is cultural and has to do with societal expectations that we be fully functional at all times. If we are anything less than this, or are in need of support and help, we may be perceived by ourselves and others as weak. When chronic pain is present, function-ing is impaired, and even though you are not being lazy, this reduced functioning may lead to inaccurate self-blaming. This then leads to the negative emotions you describe. The other reason for these negative emotions may be because your friends and family may not fully understand your pain and the attendant impairment, and then inadvertently put you down. This too can lead to these negative emotions.

Remember that chronic pain increases the risk of suf-fering from anxiety and mood disorders. As we now know, these two conditions can change our thoughts significantly in a negative direction, so this is one more issue to examine if you are facing a lot of negative emotions as you deal with chronic pain.

There is much you can do to deal with these negative emotions. First, examine your thought patterns carefully and evaluate their positive and negative characteristics. You can do this by yourself or with the help of a trusted family member, friend, or even a professional, such as your doctor or your counselor/therapist. If negative thought patterns are discovered, challenge them. Look for more adaptive and truthful thoughts, and attempt to replace the old thoughts with these new ones. If family communication is an issue, find ways to correct this (please see our specific recommendations in our response to Question 90). If you find you are suffering from depression and/or anxiety disorders, we highly recommend you find ways to address them. This issue is also discussed in more detail elsewhere in this book (please see Questions 10, 11, 39, 51, and 53). In sum-mary, negative emotions make dealing with chronic pain extra difficult. We know that negative emotions heighten pain. Work hard at pushing away negative thoughts and replace them with truthful, positive thoughts!

Sue said:

I frequently find that limited activity results in negative feelings/thoughts. I try to keep things in perspective, remembering that my pain is much improved and it's something that I have to manage. I agree that the use of cognitive (self-talk) skills is an effective way to deal with these negative thoughts.

94. What are some coping skills that can help me and my family deal better with chronic pain?

There are a large number of coping skills available to you and your loved ones as you deal with chronic pain. Here are a few for your consideration.

A positive and hopeful attitude is perhaps the top coping mechanism to have. Remember that many people before you with chronic pain have received help and have dealt with the challenges of their condition. In this way you are not alone in your suffering. Family and friends supporting you is another great coping mechanism. Being better educated about the pain condition is an excellent idea as well—knowledge is power! Optimum management of any insomnia, anxiety, or depression that you may be experiencing is another way to optimize your coping skills. Exercising to the best of your abilities is both a great emotional and physical form of enhancing your coping mechanism. Being in a support group and/or being active in your religious faith also can be wonderful coping mechanisms.

Chronic pain can often shut down lines of communication with your family and friends—do all you can to prevent this from happening. Find opportunities to connect and talk with people you love. The goal is not

Chronic pain can often shut down lines of communication with your family and friends—do all you can to prevent this from happening. Find opportunities to connect and talk with people you love.

to complain, but to derive positive energy and support from each other. Silence is not golden when it comes to dealing with chronic pain. Read more on the issue of chronic pain, which can give you both support and ideas on dealing with pain. The very fact that you are reading this book tells us you are a believer in this technique! Finally, if you run out of ideas on coping mechanisms, reach out. Talk to family, friends, professionals, clergy, support groups, or anyone who is supportive and understands your needs. There is always an undiscovered idea out there than can help you better cope with chronic pain.

Sue said:

Staying connected is so important. I always do better when I'm socially active rather than isolated. Staying active socially and physically is a great way to combat chronic pain. Learning about my difficulties has always resulted in a sense of empowerment rather than feeling like a victim.

95. What are some of the near-term breakthroughs expected in the field of pain management?

Clinicians and researchers are pouring tremendous time and energy into creating new options for people with chronic pain. As a result, treatment breakthroughs are occurring with non-medication treatment options, medication treatments, and surgical treatments. The use of cognitive-behavioral therapies (CBT) for chronic pain management has been significantly refined and can truly be considered a breakthrough in chronic pain management. Expect in the near future that your chronic pain clinicians will offer you DVDs and perhaps access to online streaming videos that will teach you enhanced CBT techniques for pain management.

Also, expect clinicians to offer you more precise information on what kinds of exercise will help you better manage your pain conditions. Pain medications are expected to become "smarter" and more precise to target your pain condition with fewer side effects as time moves forward. A huge number of pain medications are in the middle and late stages of development and will start becoming available in the next few months to years. Surgical advances are equally impressive. Less invasive techniques that target pain generating or conducting organs of the body are being studied in clinical trials. Devices to control pain are also being refined, and these devices either deliver medications for pain management, or they use electrical activity to manage pain.

We hope our enthusiasm regarding the future of pain management is coming through loud and clear. We are not being unduly optimistic; we think that we are quite appropriately positive about the future of chronic pain management. Just look at the last 25 years—the non-medication and medication treatment advances have been spectacular. The future should hold even more promise for you as a person wrestling with chronic pain. Perhaps the best way to make sure you take advantage of these emerging advances is to keep in close touch with your chronic pain management professionals and continue to ask them if new options are available to you.

96. Why is my memory not as good as it used to be since I have had chronic pain? What can I do about it?

We have heard many of our patients with chronic pain report this difficulty with memory and concentration. There is now good scientific understanding for why this might be happening to you. Pain by itself is distracting, and a person with pain is obviously focused on it and will have trouble appropriately focusing on things such as conversations, things they are reading, and so forth. In addition to this, many pain patients have disrupted sleep, which in itself harms memory and concentration. The impact of sleep on memory is so significant that pilots and truck drivers have strict rules they have to follow to avoid sleep disruptions that might affect their work. Additionally, the chemical changes that often happen during chronic pain can harm memory and sleep. Let's not forget that depression and anxiety, frequent accomplices of chronic pain, independently impair memory and concentration. We also know that chronic pain can change or damage certain parts of our brains over time, which also has adverse effects on our memory. And finally, some medication treatments for chronic pain, while helpful with the pain, can diminish memory and concentration and make you forgetful.

Although seemingly daunting, you and your clinician can work diligently to diminish the impact of memory difficulties on your life. If you personally don't notice memory problems, check with family, friends, and perhaps even coworkers to see if they notice a problem. If they do, definitely bring this up with your clinician. This may be coming from a medication that can be adjusted to diminish this problem. Or, your clinician can do a medical checkup to see if other issues, such as an undetected thyroid problem, may be a cause of your problem. Your clinician can recommend simple techniques to help you overcome memory difficulties, such as the use of notes, lists, using an electric organizer with alarms to help you, and so forth. He or she may also recommend one of several medications used to counteract memory difficulties. There are many such medications with some utility and you should discuss this issue with your clinician. Finally, be very careful driving when you are aware of a memory problem. Driving needs a great deal of attention and concentration. If you feel at all that you are an unsafe driver, we recommend you not drive until you discuss this issue with your clinician and find a solution for it. It is in your best interest, for all the reasons outlined above, to look for and treat any memory difficulties you may be facing as you attempt to conquer chronic pain.

Sue said:

I never connected my pain with memory difficulties, but it makes perfect sense. I also find that my sleep is significantly disrupted when the pain flares up. It was reassuring to understand that fragmented sleep can contribute to memory problems. The worry about memory problems is less now that I understand the connection.

97. Can complementary therapies or alternative therapies be helpful in pain management?

There are many types of complementary therapies available for the management of chronic pain. The fact that there are so many, points to the fact that many people are still not fully helped by traditional therapies and need further help. On the other hand, if you are not already engaged with a complementary therapy, you may be wondering what it is. The best definition we have found is from the National Institutes of Health (NIH) website on complementary medicine, where they offer this definition of complementary therapies: "Complementary and alternative medicine is a group of diverse medical and health care systems, practices, and products that are not generally considered part of conventional medicine."

Many Americans use complementary therapies. The National Institutes of Health estimates that 4 in 10 Americans use such therapies. Women and those of a higher socioeconomic class tend to utilize such therapies more often. Many of these complementary therapies are for pain management, including exercise, yoga, breathing exercises, and herbal products.

There are many positives and some negatives surrounding the issue of complementary medicine in pain management. Most, but not all, of these therapies have gone through at least some scientific testing either for effectiveness or safety. Often these therapies are safe, but a surprising number of times some complementary therapies have eventually proven to be problematic—at least for some people. This fact does not mean that complementary theories are to be avoided. We are proponents of patients vigorously looking into complementary therapies to find one that fits their needs, but caution must be exercised. Do your best to seek the opinions and knowledge of your health care professionals, family members, and friends. It would also be a good idea to search the Web for both positive and negative feedback. Once you choose a complementary therapy, be somewhat cautious in the beginning so that if there is a negative consequence, you can react to it appropriately.

The National Institutes of Health maintains a terrific website on complementary and alternative medicine. The NIH center involved is called NCCAM, which stands for National Center for Complementary and Alternative Medicine (www.nccam.nih.gov). The NCCAM website is loaded with great, well-balanced information. We highly recommend that you make this website an important step in your journey of exploring alternative tools as you fight your chronic pain.

98. As a chronic pain patient, does the federal government offer me any specific rights or protections?

Indeed they do! Over the last few decades, the federal government has become increasingly aware of chronic pain's impact on individuals and society at large. While pain by itself is not a federally protected issue, disability that frequently results from pain is subject to vigorous governmental oversight. If you have a pain-related disability, you should become aware of a federal act called the Americans with Disabilities Act, frequently referred to by its acronym, ADA (http://www.ada.gov/pubs/ada.htm).

This act is well understood by employers and they are under federal mandate to reasonably accommodate your disability from any cause, including chronic pain. You are advised to be aware of this act by reading up on it. We have provided a direct link above, to the language of this act from the Department of Justice. You may also discuss your needs with your employee assistance program, should one be available where you work. Also, many lawyers specialize in helping people with ADA-related conflicts with their employers. Should you have such an issue, you may want to consult a lawyer with such expertise.

Finally, the government also has a program for offering disability-related financial support to people who are temporarily or permanently disabled. Chronic pain is quite easily one of the more important issues that drive people to seek disability. Should you feel that you need such help, a great place to start the process is by visiting a very useful site—that of the U.S. Social Security Administration (http://www.socialsecurity.gov/). Look for the tab labeled "Disability," click it, and you will find a wealth of information that could be useful for your specific needs.

The federal and local governments are genuinely interested in your rights as someone afflicted with chronic pain. However, government systems are often very difficult to navigate. Thus, be patient, and get help from professionals, family members, and friends.

99. Are there any national level, pain-focused advocacy groups? I would like to join one for support, as well as help others who also have problems with pain.

There are many such organizations. It is a great idea to connect with others with similar difficulties.

There is a national chronic pain support group called, appropriately, Chronic Pain Support Group (http://www. chronicpainsupport.org/index.html). Consider checking this out.

Another organization worthy of being "checked out" is the American Chronic Pain Association (http://www. theacpa.org), whose mission is to offer peer support and education.

There also is the American Pain Foundation (http:// www.painfoundation.org), considered by many to be the best of the national level pain advocacy groups. Its website is definitely the one we recommend you visit often to get information and support.

There is a well-known advocacy group, the American Pain Society (APS) that is geared toward professionals (http://www.ampainsoc.org). While it is geared toward the medical professional, you may want to visit it to see what cutting-edge research is being conducted, as well as to be aware of legislative issues surrounding chronic pain.

You may also want to consider joining these organizations. The cause of chronic pain treatment is strengthened by your participation. Register for the free e-newsletters many of these organizations offer, and certainly consider going to meetings. All of us—professionals, patients, and their support systems (families and friends)—need to pull together to conquer chronic pain.

100. I know we have talked a lot about treating pain, but is preventing pain even a possibility? If so, what are your recommendations?

We have indeed talked a lot about treating pain, but we should discuss preventing it, thoroughly. The answer is yes, it is often possible to prevent pain.

Here is an example. If you don't take good care of your teeth by brushing them regularly, flossing, going for regular dental care, and so forth, there is a much higher likelihood you will develop tooth decay. If you develop tooth decay, then you are much more likely to have cavities and infections that are quite painful. So, here is a simple example of how preventive measures can save you from a serious source of pain—in this case, pain in your mouth.

Now, it is important for you to understand that we don't mean you can prevent every chronic pain condition. But a surprisingly large number of these pain conditions are actually quite preventable. Sometimes they are not entirely preventable, but by taking the right steps, you can delay the development of chronic pain or reduce the intensity of it.

There are many examples of this prevention approach. Here are a few that should resonate with you. If you exercise regularly, you will have stronger bones and stronger muscles. These both directly reduce the risk of chronic back pain or fractures, so you can again see how prevention works. Taking good care of your mind and body frequently prevents or reduces the risk of developing chronic pain conditions.

We advise that you take the best possible care of your body and mind before you develop any pain conditions. This is undeniably the right thing to do. Check your past and family history of chronic pain. Do you see problems with chronic pain potentially looming in the future? If so, what are they, and what preventive steps might you take? Do you need medical help to better understand this prevention plan? Do you need to take any steps right now? Remember, an ounce of prevention now is better than a pound of treatment down the road!

Glossary

A

Acupuncture: An ancient Chinese pain treatment in which needles are inserted and then manipulated along meridians where, according to Chinese texts, body energy flows.

Acute pain: Pain caused by tissue injury. Typically ceases once the injury has healed. Acute pain is an adaptive, predictable, warning signal aimed at preserving the integrity of our bodies by preventing more extensive injury to our tissues than has already been experienced.

Allodynia: Propensity to experience non-painful stimuli, such as touch and pressure, as pain. Allodynia is a common feature of many chronic pain disorders.

B

Bidirectional relationship: Reciprocal relationship. In the context of chronic pain there is an increased risk of sleep, mood, and anxiety disorders in pain sufferers, and vice versa: depression, anxiety, and sleep disturbance predict the development of widespread pain.

Body mass index (BMI): A measure based on weight and body surface, often used as an indicator of obesity.

C

Carpal tunnel syndrome (CTS): Painful condition caused by compression of a major nerve passing through a narrow space defined by carpal bones, tendons, and soft tissue. Tissue swelling will compress the nerve, causing tingling, burning, and numbness impacting the palmar side of the thumb, index finger, middle finger, and half of the ring finger.

Central sensitization: Magnified pain experience resulting from disrupted pain modulation at several levels of the central nervous system. This type of pain tends to be diffuse and generalized.

Cervical radiculopathy: Neuropathic pain due to injury of the cervical nerve roots, most often caused by compression. Commonly manifests as pain in the neck and one arm, and is associated with weakness and a loss of sensation in the area affected by nerve-root distribution.

Chronic Fatigue Syndrome (CFS): A prolonged medical condition of unknown cause, characterized by a sensation of exhaustion, inability to carry out physical and intellectual tasks, fever, aches, and depression.

Chronic pain: Persists in the absence of an ongoing stimulus, well beyond the resolution of the underlying disease, sometimes lasting for months or even years.

Cluster headaches: Characterized by clearly delineated pain attacks in the innervation area of the first branch of the trigeminal nerve impacting the areas around the eye socket and forehead.

Cognitive-behavioral therapy (CBT): Originally developed to help treat patients with depression, this therapy teaches patients to harness the power of their thoughts and change their behaviors to improve their mood and functioning.

Comorbidity: An accompanying condition to a previous illness.

Complex Regional Pain Syndrome (CRPS): A combined inflammatory and neuropathic pain disorder, which usually develops after a limb injury. This condition is characterized by excessive pain (hyperalgesia), tenderness to touch (allodynia), tingling and numbness, sweaty, flushed, skin of abnormal temperature, and impairment of motion.

Corticosteroids: A group of steroid hormones produced by the cortex of the adrenal gland or made synthetically. These "stress" hormones typically have anti-inflammatory and immunosuppressant properties.

COX-2 inhibitors: Medications designed to inhibit cyclooxygenase-2, an enzyme involved in synthesis of prostaglandins. These agents have anti-inflammatory and analgesic (painkiller) properties.

D

Diabetic neuropathy (DNP): Condition caused by injury to the nerves, most likely due to microvascular disease. Small blood vessels supplying nerves are occluded due to diabetes and can no longer fulfill their role. It is characterized by pain described as sharp, stinging, burning, aching, or electrical. Typically associated with numbness and tingling, loss of sensation to temperature, pressure, or pain.

F

Fibromyalgia (FM): Characterized by chronic widespread pain (tenderness in at least 11 of 18 predefined points on the surface of the body), lasting at least 3 months, typically accompanied by fatigue and sleep disturbance.

"First pain": Initial pain experience produced by activation of myelinated A-delta type pain fibers. Commonly described as sharp, stabbing, and well-defined.

H

Hyperalgesia: A tendency to experience painful stimuli as much more intense than they really are.

Hypothalamic–pituitary–adrenal (HPA) axis: Neuroendocrine system composed of several interrelated components (hypothalamus, pituitary, and adrenal glands). Complex regulatory feedback loops optimize the levels of stress hormones, including cortisol, adreno-corticotropic hormone (ACTH), and corticotropin-releasing hormone (CRH). The HPA axis is involved in the regulation of diverse processes, such as energy expenditure, immune function, sexuality, digestion, and mood.

I

Inflammatory pain: Arises in response to infection, tissue damage, or irritation. When our bodies are exposed to injurious stimuli, they commonly generate an "inflammatory soup," which is a mix of chemicals produced by the injured tissue and our immune cells. This mix includes ions, bradykinins, pro-inflammatory cytokines, prostaglandins, and other chemicals. "Inflammatory soup" washes over sensory nerve endings and produces inflammatory pain as a signal warning us that our bodies are under invasion.

Intrathecal pump therapy: Treatment based on the delivery of pain medication directly into the cerebrospinal fluid via a small medical device.

Irritable bowel syndrome (IBS): Chronic functional digestive disorder characterized by recurrent abdominal pain, relieved by defecation, and accompanied by disturbance of bowel habits, bloating, and discomfort in the absence of an identifiable organic cause.

L

Learned helplessness: As a result of physical (chronic pain), or emotional adversities (sexual abuse, physical or mental abuse, depression, anxiety, and/or stress), a person comes to believe that things will never get better. Consequently, feelings of helplessness may progress and solidify into a constant belief system.

Low back pain (LBP): Pain that originates from spinal ligaments, facet joints, the periosteum, paravertebral muscles, fascia, and compressed spinal nerve roots. Most commonly, the pain is of musculoskeletal origin related to the degeneration of facet joints and intervertebral disks.

M

Meditation: A contemplative process whereby an individual attempts to get beyond reflexive thinking into a state of more profound awareness and relaxation.

Migraine headaches: Neurobiological condition characterized by unilateral throbbing headaches, accompanied by nausea, vomiting, and hypersensitivity to light and sound. Migraines affect women much more frequently than men.

Multiple sclerosis (MS): An immune-mediated neurological disorder that typically follows a relapsing-remitting course. The disease typically starts with sensory disturbances, double vision, limb weakness, clumsiness, gait disturbance, fatigue, and neurogenic bladder and bowel problems. Eventually, cognitive and emotional problems, including affective lability, vertigo, pain, and widespread loss of strength and sensation, may develop.

Myofascial pain: A chronic condition associated with localized muscle stiffness and pain (often severe); palpable hypersensitive nodules in muscle tissue, often referred to as "trigger points"; referred tenderness and pain; and motor and autonomic dysfunction. It is believed to be based on central sensitization.

N

Nerve blocks: Injection of local anesthetic in vicinity of nerves for temporary control of pain.

Neuropathic pain (NeP): Typically caused by direct nerve injury or dysfunction of the neural tissue, resulting in abnormal sensory processing.

Nociceptive pain: Pain caused by tissue injury. Pain is due to mechanical, thermal, or chemical injury to bodily tissue. Diverse painful stimuli are converted by nociceptors (sensory nerve endings) into an electrochemical signal, which is then propagated to the dorsal horn of the spinal column and eventually to the pain-processing circuitry in the brain, providing us with a comprehensive pain experience.

Nociceptors: Specialized pain-sensing nerve endings that detect chemical, mechanical, or thermal injury to our tissues.

Norepinephrine: A catecholamine (type of monoamine) synthesized from dopamine. Norepinephrine may act as a hormone, when secreted into the bloodstream from the adrenal medulla, or as a neurotransmitter in the central nervous system and sympathetic nervous system where it is released by noradrenergic nerve endings. The actions of norepinephrine are carried out via the binding to adrenergic receptors. Norepinephrine has a principal role in the fight-or-flight response, directly increasing heart rate, triggering the release of glucose from energy stores, and increasing blood flow to skeletal muscles, the heart, and brain.

NSAIDs: Abbreviation designating nonsteroidal anti-inflammatory drugs; medications with analgesic (pain-reducing) and antipyretic (fever-reducing) properties. Higher doses also have anti-inflammatory activity (reducing inflammation).

O

Opioids: Medications and substances generated by our brain cells that attach themselves to receptors on the cell membranes, that specifically respond to them. Opioids are centuries-old medications, and if derived from a plant they are called natural, but they can also be semi-synthetic or synthetic. Opioids are powerful pain medications and unfortunately also common drugs of abuse. Endogenous opioids are created by our brain cells and play a roll in the regulation of pain, stress response, and mood.

Osteoarthritis (OA): A painful condition of the joints, particularly affecting us with increasing age. Characterized by the following abnormalities: (1) damage to joint cartilage and subchondral bone, centered on weight bearing areas, (2) inflammation and thickening of the joint capsule, (3) aberrant bone formation at the joint margins (osteophytes), and (4) inflammation of synovial membranes.

P

Pain: An unpleasant sensory, emotional, and cognitive experience generated in response to actual or potential tissue injury.

Paresthesia: Altered feeling of pain that can affect any nerve(s) in the body. Patients typically report burning and/or tingling pain.

Peripheral sensitization: Painful signals continue to flow from the periphery to dorsal column, long after the harmful stimulus has stopped or to a degree that is excessively out of proportion to the magnitude of the original source of pain.

Phantom limb pain (PLP): Localized predominantly in the distal part of the missing limb. For example, if the lower limb has been amputated, pain will be experienced in the area where the toes, heel, ankle, and instep were, even though they are no longer attached to the person's body.

Physical medicine and rehabilitation (PMR): A medical specialty, practiced by physicians who are exceptionally well-trained in helping patients with limitations imposed by strokes, head injuries, cardiovascular disease, muscle, bone, joint and soft tissue injury. Physical medicine specialists have significant expertise in helping patients with chronic pain.

Placebo: A dummy pill (most often starch) that does not contain the medication; it is often used in controlled trials for new medications.

Plantar fasciitis: An inflammation of the ligaments in the foot, characterized by a sharp, stabbing pain in the heel of the foot upon taking the first few steps after awakening.

Post-herpetic neuralgia (PHN): A painful condition caused by nerve damage after a person experiences shingles (also called herpes zoster). This can happen even after the skin lesions have disappeared.

Proctalgia fugax: Characterized by fleeting, paroxysmal pain of the rectal/anal area.

Proctodynia: Characterized by pain in the rectal/anal area of the body.

Prostatodynia: A common urogenital pain disorder of unknown origin, typically occurring in men between the ages of 20 to 60 years. Patients suffering from prostatodynia often complain of pain during urination, urinary urgency followed by poor urinary flow, and pain in the pelvic floor.

R

Radiating pain: Pain felt in parts of the body where there is no cause of pain. Often caused by a "pinched," squeezed, or damaged nerve elsewhere. For example, a person can feel pain that shoots down the legs or buttocks even when the damage is in the pelvic region.

Rheumatoid arthritis (RA): An autoimmune disorder (when "confused" immune system turns against our own tissue, "mistaking" it for a foreign substance) characterized by chronic inflammation of multiple joints, associated with destruction of cartilage and adjoining bony structures.

S

Serotonin: A monoamine neurotransmitter (a chemical substance the brain and the body uses to help transmit information between nerves) involved with multiple bodily functions, including digestion, blood clotting, temperature, mood and anxiety regulation.

Spinal stenosis: Caused by narrowing of the central spinal canal or lateral recesses, most often due to age-related hypertrophy of joint facets or thickening of ligamentum flavum, either of which cause compression of the spinal cord and the nerves.

Spondylitis: Inflamed or degenerated joints between different vertebrae in the spine. Symptoms include leg pain after walking, tingling, and numbness.

Steroids: Both natural and synthetic chemicals that have different effects on the body. Natural steroids are essential for healthy living, and too much or too little can cause major problems. Steroids help people deal with stress and modulate inflammation and immune responses. Chronic pain disorders are often associated with irregular steroid activity.

T

Tarsal tunnel syndrome (TTS): A painful neuropathic condition caused by compression of the posterior tibial nerve in the tarsal tunnel, which is a part of the foot where ligaments form a space (a tunnel) through which this nerve travels. When the tunnel is narrowed, the nerve is compressed, causing pain.

Temporal summation of "second pain" (TSSP): This is a complex response whereby pain fibers, when continuously stimulated by pain or inflammation, "learn to over-feel" pain. Intensity of pain is out of proportion with the actual injury, and patients often report dull, aching, burning, and diffuse, spread-out pain. TSSP is associated with elevated activity in several brain pain-processing areas.

Temporomandibular joint (TMJ) pain disorders: The jaw bone is connected to the skull with a hinge joint. When this joint degenerates or becomes inflamed, a person can experience facial pain, limited motion, or stiffness in the muscles of the lower jaw, and crackling sounds while making chewing motions. Additionally, patients will often complain of headaches, pain and buzzing in their ears, dizziness, and neck pain.

Tolerance: A pharmacological phenomenon in which a person who takes a certain dose of medication on a regular basis notices a gradual decrease in benefits derived from the medication.

Trigger points: Specific points in our body that, when irritated, cause pain in other parts of the body. Doctors will often look for these points to inject pain medication in order to reduce pain.

V

Vulvodynia: A chronic pain syndrome lasting at least 3 months manifested by vulvar (external female genitalia) discomfort, burning and/or stinging pain, irritation, and dyspareunia (painful or uncomfortable intercourse).

Index

H

headaches
    cluster, 29–30
    deadly, 25–26
    migraine, 28–29
    severe, 27
    tension, 12
health, cellular/subcellular, 84
helplessness, learned, 80–81
hematoma
    epidural, 25
    intraparenchymal, 25
    subdural, 26
hemorrhage, subarachnoid, 26–28
herpes zoster virus, 42–43
hippocampus, 15–16
hormone regulation, 21
HPA axis. *See* hypothalamic-pituitary-
        adrenal axis
hyperalgesia, 9–10, 37, 66
hypothalamic-pituitary-adrenal axis
        (HPA axis), 56
    chronic pain and, 69–70
    definition of, 69
    role of, 72–73
hypothalamus, 16
hypoxia, 30

I

IBS. *See* irritable bowel syndrome
ibuprofen, 97
IC. *See* insular cortex
IL-8. *See* interleukin-8
imaging studies, for back pain, 131–132
immune regulation, sleep and, 19
immunity, chronic pain and, 72–74
indomethacin, 97
infection, 3
inflammation
    chemical mediators of, 8
    chronic pain and, 71
    DNP and, 46
    increases in, 73–74
    meditation and, 85
    reduction of, 118
    sleep deprivation and, 19
inflammatory pain, 2–3
"inflammatory soup," 3, 6
inhibitory pathways, 46–47, 66
insomnia, 18
insula, 66
insular cortex (IC), 7, 16
interleukin-8 (IL-8), 74

interstitial cystitis, 12
intraparenchymal hematoma, 25
intrathecal pump therapy, medications and,
        128–129
irritable bowel syndrome (IBS), 12
    aggravation of, 48–49
    causes of, 49
    classifications of, 47
    definition of, 47
    pain and, 47–49

K

ketoprofen, 97
kindling, 14

L

LBP. *See* low back pain
learned helplessness, 80–81
Lewis, Jerry, 129–130
lidocaine patches, 97
limbic function, changes in, 15
limbic system, activation of, 63
liver failure, 115
low back pain (LBP)
    acute, 32
    causes of, 31–33
    definition of, 31
    diagnosis of, 33–35
    imaging studies for, 131–132
    nerve stimulator for, 129–130
    recurrence of, 33

M

major depressive disorders, 16; *See also*
        depression
    neurotransmitter abnormalities and, 60
marijuana, pain management and, 116–117
medial malleolus, 40
medial prefrontal cortex (mPFC), 67
median nerve, 39
medications, 96–98; *See also* opioids; over-
        the-counter medications
    addictive potential of, 110–111
    anticonvulsant, 97
    antidepressant, 97–100
    antiseizure, 111–112
    anti-epileptic, 97, 111–112
    in combination, 104, 106–108
    for epilepsy, 97, 111–112
    FDA-approval of, 101–102
    half life of, 103
    illegally diverted/obtained, 105
    intrathecal pump therapy and, 128–129
    long-term use of, 115–116

Index

JUN - - 2011

Northport-East Northport Public Library

To view your patron record from a computer, click on
the Library's homepage: **www.nenpl.org**

You may:
- request an item be placed on hold
- renew an item that is overdue
- view titles and due dates checked out on your card
- view your own outstanding fines

**151 Laurel Avenue
Northport, NY 11768
631-261-6930**